A Guide to

Improving Food Hygiene

Graham Aston and John Tiffney

Northwood Publications Ltd
London EC1V 7QA

Published 1977

ISBN 7198 2644 6

A 'Catering Times' book

Typeset by Bacchus Ltd, London
Printed and bound in Great Britain by The Grange Press, Southwick, Sussex.

CONTENTS

PREFACE

The aim of this book is to try impart some of the basic rules of clean food handling to the large number of people engaged in the food industry. We have tried to write the book in plain language in the hope that everyone, from the kitchen porter to supermarket manager, will find something of interest. For those readers who wish to further their knowledge, we have provided a bibliography of reference books at the end of the book.

It is a fact that the catering industry of Britain is a major stable industry with a turnover of £1,500 million a year. Every weekday more than 22 million meals or snacks are served outside the home. About 7 million people buy food in hotels, restaurants, take-aways, pubs, cafes, snack bars and wine bars; 6 million meals are eaten in industrial and commercial premises; 7.4 million meals are served in schools and educational establishments; and 1.9 million meals in hospitals and other institutions. With such a large number of people eating out each day, it is essential to ensure that the food being served is of the highest quality. This brings us back to the reason why we wrote the book, quite simply we thought that there was a need to publish a guide to hygienic food handling.

"Prevention is better than cure" is a well-known proverb which aptly fits this subject. Food poisoning results in illness and even death can affect hundreds of people in a single outbreak caused by one careless food handler. Quite apart from the personal suffering and inconvenience, the loss of production and earnings can cost the country many millions of pounds a year. If better food handling reduces this risk of infection and expense, then a significant contribution will have been made to the nation's health and wealth. This book endeavours to identify simple, inexpensive methods and materials which can forestall the conditions most likely to produce food poisoning. Investing and indulging in these principles should reap the rewards of continued and increasing public confidence in your establishment or enterprise.

Thankfully, it is pleasing to note that more interest is being taken in the subject of food hygiene and various organisations are playing a major role in training those in the industry. The Royal Society of Health, the Environmental Health Officers' Association in conjunction with St. John's Ambulance, the Hotel and Catering Industry Training Board and the Hospital Caterers' Association are all involved with food hygiene training and this book has been designed to cater for the needs of students attending their courses. We hope too that others with a lesser though nonetheless important involvement with the subject will derive some benefit from reading it. Domestic science teachers, nurses, doctors and housewives should all be able to find something of value.

We would like to thank the following people for their contributions towards making this book possible: our secretaries Peg and Pauline for their forebearance and cheerful typing under the severest provocation; our wives Karen and Linda for becoming "book widows" while we scribbled; Mr Peter Bateman and other staff at Rentokil Ltd for their kind assistance and the many companies who have supplied photographs. Finally, we wish to record our thanks to our respective authorities for their interest in the project.

GRAHAM ASTON
JOHN TIFFNEY

June 1977

INTRODUCTION

The subject of food hygiene has existed from the time when man realised for the first time that unless he handled his food in a certain way he would be ill. Today the lessons that he learned by trial and error still form the basis for good practice by food handlers in their work.

We know from earlier writings that man realised that food kept better when in cool surroundings and that unclean hands could contaminate food to make people ill. We know too that eating certain animals and birds was frowned upon because they had long been associated with illness and although the precise reasons for the illness were unknown, early man began to understand for himself that good sound food, properly prepared, was essential to good health.

The need for food hygiene has increased over the years and has been influenced by a number of factors. The earlier influence, of course, was the knowledge that unsound or ill-handled food could cause illness. But in small communities where each family produced and cooked its own food, the effect of poor handling was confined to the family. On a larger scale there are records of early communal feedings by armies where more soldiers had been put down by the food they ate than by the slings and arrows of the enemy. It is a recognised fact that in war time today amongst the most vulnerable features are the food and water supplies.

Communal feeding in the early days probably gave rise to an increased interest in food hygiene for careless handling by one person could suddenly affect a great number of people. The industrial revolution in this country saw for the first time a great influx from the country to the larger towns or newly founded industrial centres and as these people needed to be housed, so they needed to be fed. Books of the period illustrate clearly the squalor of living conditions and the associated diseases. The lack of proper drainage, refuse disposal, clean air and water supplies all contributed to a dismal picture, but whilst all this was going on, people were being fed in equally appalling conditions and by those with neither experience nor expertise. There is no doubt that food poisoning was common and resulted in many deaths and an overwhelming amount of general sickness.

Doctors of the day, of course, had little knowledge of diagnosis and lacked the laboratory facilities for testing that we have today but we can see from early records that many of the reasons for deaths were probably no more than different names for the same condition, namely food poisoning. "Collick and winde, griping of the guts and rising of the lights (vomiting)" are all conditions that accounted for many deaths in the early days and as these all appear to be associated with the alimentary canal, it is fair to assume that unsound food was probably the cause.

From the simple experiments by Louis Pasteur, who proved that those invisible organisms or bacteria that caused spoilage could be killed by the application of heat, there emerged a whole new scientific approach to the preservation of food. The process of pasteurisation stands as a memorial to the French scientist. It has no doubt done more to ensure the safety of our food than any other single development. Later, the introduction of laboratory techniques to grow and isolate different types of bacteria and the development of more sophisticated microscopes gave man the means by which he could now identify those invisible enemies, thereby making the task of controlling them much easier.

Today, in this country, legislation exists to help to prevent food poisoning and those who subject the consumer to risk can be punished. The fact remains that food poisoning continues to cause considerable illness and because of this an efficient system operates to deal with cases once they arise.

The general practitioner will diagnose what he believes to be food poisoning. Specimens from the patient will probably be submitted to one of the many Public Health Laboratories for examination. These laboratories form a network throughout the country and are staffed by specialist chemists and bacteriologists who have the facilities to confirm and identify the type of poisoning. Once confirmation of the poisoning is given, the general practitioner is then able to embark upon a course of treatment to restore the patient to health.

While all the tests are being carried out, the Environmental Health

Officer will have started his investigations to try and find out the source of the poisoning. It may be that the patient visited a particular restaurant or café and ate unsound food. It may be that a number of people are affected — or it may just be a case of a housewife forgetting the basic requirements of food hygiene.

After a thorough investigation often involving very many people being interviewed, the Environmental Health Officer would hope finally to identify the cause. What is most important is that he will then seek to ensure that the source is eliminated.

Unfortunately, most cases of food poisoning arise through carelessness and on occasion it is not possible to isolate the cause of the sickness. Nonetheless the Environmental Health Officer will doubtless take the opportunity to question food handlers about their method of operation to see if there is room for improvement.

Success invariably comes from a better understanding . . . now read on.

Chapter 1

THE LAW AND THE FOOD TRADE

The principal Act of Parliament governing the food trade is the Food & Drugs Act, 1955, which makes stipulations concerning the storage, manufacture and sale of all foodstuffs and provides for Regulations to be made to provide detailed guidance on, for example, colouring matter, preservatives and the composition of food. Every person involved in food manufacturing should be conversant with the legal requirements of the country. Since joining the European Economic Community, there have been progressive moves to "harmonise" the legislation of the various nations and it is apparent that food manufacturers have had to comply with member states' food laws in order to export their products successfully.

Our principal interest lies in the legislation in England and Wales concerning food hygiene standards in food premises, and inevitably this leads us in a number of different directions.

The Food & Drug Act, 1955, stipulates the following requirements:

1. The appropriate Ministers may take regulations for the protection of the public health in food premises. Regulations have been made to cover a number of important aspects of food handling. (See later notes)
2. A local authority must register, if thought suitable, premises used for the storage, manufacture and sale of ice-cream, and the preparation or manufacture of potted, pressed, pickled or preserved food and sausages. Catering premises, schools and clubs are exempted from these conditions.

3. Every ice-cream vendor who sells ice-cream in a street or public place must display his name and address.
4. Every ice-cream manufacturer or dealer must notify the local authority if he knows that any food handler is suffering from one of the following infectious diseases: typhoid, para-typhoid, dysentery, diptheria, scarlet fever, gastro-enteritis, undulant fever, throat infection.
5. A registered medical practitioner must notify the local authority if he becomes aware or suspects that a patient is suffering from food poisoning.
6. If a local authority officer suspects that any food is liable to cause food poisoning, he may prohibit the use of the food for human consumption until his investigations are completed.
7. An authorised officer of a local authority shall, on producing on request some duly authenticated document, have a right of entry into any premises at all reasonable times.

The Food and Drugs (Control of Food Premises) Act, 1976, gives local authorities in England and Wales powers to apply to a Magistrate's Court for a Closure Order to be made in respect of any food business operating from fixed premises or a stall. The local authority must give the owner of the business notice of its intention to apply to the Court for an Order and the Court must hear representations from the authority and the owner in order to decide whether the condition of the premises presents a risk of danger to health sufficient to justify making such an order. The order remains in force until the local authority certify that the danger to health has been removed. The Act also makes provision for a court to issue an Emergency Order in cases where the continuing use of a food premises presents an imminent risk to health. Appeal procedures against the court decision and in relation to compensation for loss of business are specified.

This procedure will only be used by local authorities in extreme cases where all normal methods of education and persuasion have failed.

The Food Hygiene (General) Regulations, 1970, are of prime importance to everyone engaged in the food trade, and a copy of the Regulations should be available for all to read. Staff should be given instruction on their obligations to ensure clean food production whilst remembering that these Regulations only prescribe a minimum standard. Many food premises and their staff maintain a far higher standard of hygiene which sets a target for the remainder to try to achieve. It is hoped that the following notes will serve as a guide to the Regulations.

1. The Regulations apply to all premises where food is manufactured, stored or sold, whether for profit or not; it would therefore be impossible to list all the various classes of business trading, but they would range from the public house to the staff canteen, or the sports club pavilion to the supermarket or school. Slaughterhouses, mobile traders, stalls, docks and shipping have separate regulations governing them, as detailed later in this chapter.

2. The premises in which food is handled must be clean and in good condition. There must be no risk of contamination by dirt, germs, insects, rodents, odours or in any other way.

3. The walls, floors, ceilings, windows, doors and equipment must be properly constructed and maintained in a sound condition to enable a high standard of cleanliness to be attained at all times.

4. All parts of the premises must be efficiently lighted and ventilated.

5. Sufficient sinks with hot and cold running water must be provided to enable food and equipment to be thoroughly washed. Similarly all premises must have sufficient washhand basins conveniently situated to enable staff to maintain a high standard of personal hygiene. Such basins must be supplied with hot and cold running water, soap, clean towels (or other means of drying) and nail brushes, kept clean and not used for any other purpose.

6. The water supply to the premises should be clean and wholesome — i.e., a mains supply.

7. Adequate sanitary conveniences must be provided for use by the staff and drainage systems should be in perfect working order. Refuse and waste food should be properly stored and regularly removed.

8. Staff should wear suitable clean protective clothing to avoid any risk of contamination and lockers or cupboards provided to accommodate staff outdoor clothing. First aid facilities, waterproof dressings, antiseptics and bandages should be available at all times in case of accidents.

9. Above all, staff should not smoke or engage in any unhygienic practice; food should be covered to protect it from risk of contamination and should be stored at the correct temperature to avoid the risk of food poisoning. This is especially true of foods such as meat, cooked meats, gravy, eggs, cream and dairy products.

10. Animals should not be allowed in food premises; food should not be placed within 0.5 metres (18 inches) of the floor in any forecourt or yard. Pet food or food not intended for human consumption should not

be kept in a food room unless in a closed container.

The local authority, through their Environmental Health Officers, are responsible for the enforcement of these regulations and advice should be sought on any aspect of the legislation, particularly the interpretation of the rules when alterations to premises are being considered. In recent years local authorities have been taking a tough line with proprietors of unhygienic food businesses and the Courts have imposed heavy fines to emphasise the seriousness of any failure to observe these basic regulations.

The Food Hygiene (Docks, Carriers, etc.) Regulations, 1960, govern the hygiene of food in docks, warehouses, cold stores and carrier's premises, and closely follow the General Regulations already described.

The Food Hygiene (Markets, Stalls and Delivery Vehicles) Regulations, 1966.
As the name implies, these Regulations concern the hygienic handling of food in covered markets, stalls in open air markets or streets and forecourts, and food delivery vehicles (with certain exceptions). The Regulations closely follow the General Regulations in respect of the personal hygiene rules for food handlers; i.e., clean washable clothing, first aid facilities, infectious disease control, no smoking or spitting.

All stalls and delivery vehicles must display the name and address of the owner of the business in a prominent position.

All stalls, vehicles and equipment must be kept clean, well maintained and properly lighted, and there should be no risk of contamination of food on or around the stall. The stall must be covered on the top and three sides for this reason.

There should be adequate supplies of hot and cold running water at sinks and washhand basins, soap, towels and nail brushes, although these can be provided on a communal basis if the local authority approves. Stalls selling roast chestnuts or hot potatoes are exempt from these particular requirements, as are fruiterers and greengrocers stalls from providing sinks if they are registered with the local authority.

Bread delivery vans are exempt from the provision of washhand basins, sinks and first aid facilities, as are vehicles carrying only covered or wrapped food, if they operate from or between premises where these facilities exist and are readily available to the personnel.

Vehicles used for carrying meat must be specially constructed to prevent contamination, and meat must not touch the floor. Offal must be carried in watertight receptacles and kept separate from any meat. Any person carrying meat must wear suitable headgear to prevent contamination.

These Regulations are also enforced by the Environmental Health Officers of the local authority; failure to comply with the requirements could lead to a prosecution in the Magistrates' Court with fines of up to £100 for each conviction.

Milk & Dairies (General) Regulations, 1959

These Regulations govern the hygienic production of milk and are principally concerned with dairies on farms which are the responsibility of the Ministry of Agriculture, Fisheries & Food. The requirements relate to the hygiene of personnel, premises and equipment used in milk production and storage at the dairy farm, at the dairy or bottling plant and at the retail shop.

In the latter cases the Regulations are enforced by the local authority and all shops must be registered to sell milk, although this is of far less use than in the days of untreated milk which was sold "loose" from the churn. Any person who works or resides at a dairy or dairy farm and who believes that he or a member of his household is suffering from a notifiable infectious disease, must notify the local authority whose proper officer is empowered to prohibit the use of such milk for human consumption until satisfied that any risk of infection is over.

Law and the meat trade

The slaughtering of animals for the red meat trade has been the subject of separate legislation in this country for many years. It is a sobering thought however, that it has only been possible to demand comprehensive inspection of meat and offal for human consumption since 1964. Prior to that year the service depended upon co-operation between the trade and the local authorities, but today no meat intended for human consumption can leave the abattoir or slaughterhouse until it has been inspected and stamped as being fit for human consumption. Special provisions exist for dealing with unfit meat or offal, which must be heat-treated before use as animal food.

Before the Second World War, there were some 3,000 slaughter-houses of varying sizes in England and Wales, but these were reduced to some 1,400 by 1952, when the Ministry of Food finally removed the wartime restrictions. Today the figure is approximately 1,500 slaughter-houses but, with the impact of the E.E.C., it is anticipated that many will close as production is concentrated in larger, purpose-built abattoirs.

The Slaughterhouses Act, 1974

This Act requires local authorities to issue annual licences to slaughterhouses in their districts and to supervise the operating standards and conditions under which meat is prepared for sale. The Act also regulates the use of licensed knacker's yards where animals, including horses, are slaughtered but the flesh is not intended for human consumption. Slaughtermen must also be licensed annually by the local authority, and the slaughtering of animals must be carried out in a humane way to avoid suffering. Special arrangements are allowed for Jewish and Muslim methods of slaughter.

The Slaughterhouses (Hygiene) Regulations, 1958

These Regulations govern the hygiene of slaughterhouse premises and personnel. The entire operation from the lairage accommodation of live animals to the inspection of the carcase and offal, and handling and storage of by-products such as hides and skins, has to be carried out in a clean manner, ensuring no risk of contamination. In many ways the regulations correspond to the Food Hygiene (General) Regulations, 1970, but with specific references to the various operations of a slaughterhouse such as the provision of satisfactory facilities for meat inspection. Adequate ventilation and lighting are required and minimum standards are specified for lighting in the slaughterhall and workrooms. The provision of suitable sanitary accommodation, washing facilities and first aid equipment is specified. Personal hygiene rules are similar to those for all other food handlers dealing with protective clothing, hand-washing, use of tobacco, notification of infectious diseases and avoiding contamination of blood or meat. New regulations will be introduced in 1978.

Slaughter of Animals (Prevention of Cruelty) Regulations, 1958

These Regulations are designed to ensure that any animal destined for slaughter is protected from unnecessary suffering whilst confined to a lairage or immediately prior to being slaughtered.

Both sets of Regulations are administered by the local authority through their Environmental Health Department, and offences can be punished with substantial fines on each conviction.

Slaughter of Poultry Act, 1967

This Act requires that all turkeys and domestic fowl intended for human consumption must be slaughtered instantaneously. If stunning is employed prior to slaughter, the premises must be registered with the local authority. The primary purpose of the Act is to prevent cruelty.

Poultry Meat (Hygiene) Regulations, 1976

These Regulations were introduced as part of the E.E.C. harmonisation programme and sought to provide a system of inspection for poultry meat along similar lines to red meat. The poultry industry grew to mammoth proportions during the 1960s and 1970s and considerable concern had been expressed over the lack of any significant supervision of the trade other than that exercised by the responsible producers themselves. Poultry suffer from a variety of diseases, notably salmonellosis, which are transmissible to man. Because of the capital investment required to bring the majority of premises up to the specified standard and the obligations on local authorities to train new poultry meat inspectors to carry out the inspection procedures, the full impact of the Regulations was phased over two years. They come fully into force on 15 August 1979. The exemption in respect of sales of uneviscerated poultry direct from farms lasts until August 1981, when it is to be reviewed. The Regulations require all poultry slaughterhouses to be licensed by the local authority and enables it to recover the cost of providing the inspection service. The premises and personnel must comply with the hygiene standards specified in the Regulations, which are similar to those for all food premises.

Future Legislation

Predicting the future trends in legislation governing food and food premises is an unenviable task, but it is likely that the Food & Drugs Act, 1955, will be brought up to date to reflect more recent trends in technology such as frozen foods, microwave ovens, vacuum packing and the like. The greatest influence will be that of the E.E.C. and the progressive harmonisation of the legislation between the Member States to obtain identical standards governing composition and quality of individual food products in particular. Common food hygiene rules may present difficulties and indeed may not serve any useful purpose, because they are only intended to protect the consumer in the home country except when related to food produced for export. The major difficulty is that only Great Britain and Sweden have Environmental Health Officers carrying out specific food hygiene duties, whereas other European countries use chemists, veterinary officers and even police officers.

While the Department of Health and Social Security, the Ministry of Agriculture, Fisheries and Food, and the various trade-sponsored research Institutes are all hard at work developing and assessing new methods, machinery and materials, there is no co-ordinated effort aimed at improving the standard of catering premises and equipment. An attempt has been made to produce a British Standards Institute Code of Practice for Catering Premises and Equipment, but this requires investment and extensive preparation prior to publication. It is to be applauded as a long overdue step in the right direction.

One cannot therefore over-emphasise that the present legal standards are merely a bare minimum guide, and all personnel and premises should set and achieve far higher standards at all times.

The following legislation applies to commercial and industrial premises, including food businesses, and makes provision for the health and welfare of staff (see Chapter 10).

The Factories Act, 1961, and The Offices, Shops, & Railway Premises Act, 1963

Section 9: Suitable and sufficient sanitary conveniences must be provided for staff in accordance with the Sanitary Conveniences Regulations, 1964 (below). The conveniences must be kept clean and properly maintained, with effective lighting and ventilation.

Section 10: Suitable and sufficient washing facilities must be provided for staff use, including a supply of clean, running hot and cold water or warm water, and soap and clean towels or other effective means of cleaning and drying. The Washing Facilities Regulations, 1964, identify standards for the provision of these facilities.

Chapter 2

FOOD POISONING

Food poisoning has been recognised as a disease of man since the days of Hippocrates (460-377 B.C.). Murder by poisoning was rife during the Roman Empire, oysters being a popular vehicle for removing the unwanted. In the Middle Ages poisoning was so common that official food tasters were familiar members of all Royal Courts. The sale of diseased and contaminated food was commonplace until the introduction of sanitary measures during the nineteenth century. These were slowly developed at the end of the last century and the early part of this century into the food inspection and hygiene system we operate in Britain today.

In order to understand the different types of food poisoning, particularly of a bacterial origin, it is necessary to examine the basic fundamentals of bacteriology. Bacteria or germs in the popular sense of the word are an essential part of human life, as we could not live without them. Many bacteria are harmless, and indeed some are necessary in certain processes. Examples of this are in the treatment of sewage and the production of cheese, beer and yoghurt. Those which are responsible for causing illness are called pathogenic bacteria.

Bacteria differ in shape, size and habitat but unfortunately are invisible except under a powerful microscope; it is therefore impossible to identify the source of an infection either quickly or easily. Bacteria need certain conditions in which to thrive, namely:—

1. correct temperature;
2. humidity;
3. food or media on which to feed; and
4. time to multiply.

TEMPERATURE . . . TIME . . .

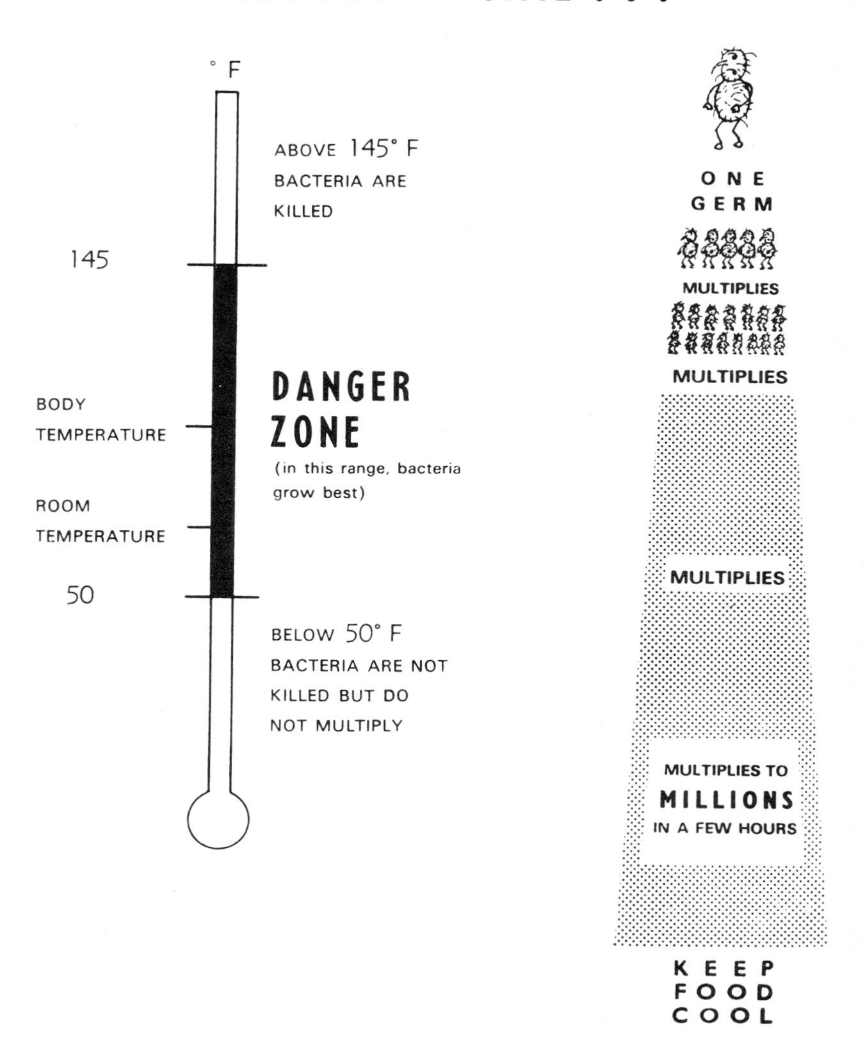

KEEP
FOOD
COOL

There are types of bacteria which like cold temperatures, ambient temperatures and even temperatures up to 75°C (167°F) but none survive the entire range. It is a common but erroneous belief that cold temperatures will kill bacteria — they are merely slowed down! Exposure to heat, on the other hand, will kill bacteria provided a sufficiently high temperature is maintained for long enough. Moisture is essential to all bacteria as their outer cell protoplasm contains a high percentage of water. This explains why the primitive method of preserving food was to dry it. All bacteria need food in some form, such as blood, serum, dirt, meat, eggs, etc. Bacteria can be classified according to their chemical status: i.e. whether they prefer acid, alkaline or neutral environments in which to live. Most bacteria thrive on acidic (meat and fruit) or neutral food substances. Finally, most bacteria dislike light, especially ultra violet light (radiation from the sun or artificially induced).

In ideal conditions most bacteria can double their numbers every 20 minutes and reach several million in 24 hours. That is the main reason for taking all possible precautions to keep the contamination to a minimum by proper hygienic measures, and to minimise opportunities for microbial growth. The process of multiplication by dividing into two is known as binary fission.

Unfortunately some pathogenic bacteria can survive for up to 14 weeks out of contact with the human or animal body — just lying in dust or floating in the air. There are also certain bacteria which can produce spores which are particularly resistant. Tetanus and anthrax, for example, can live for several hundred years in the soil.

Harmful bacteria are capable of producing poisons or toxins which cause illness in humans. Some bacteria produce the toxins outside their own cells (exotoxins) so that they mix with the surroundings. While they can be particularly lethal, heat readily kills them with the important exception of *Staphylococcus exotoxin*. On the other hand, endotoxins are produced within the bacterial cell and are not usually released until the germ dies. These endotoxins are more resistant to heat and tend to take much longer to cause illness because it takes longer for sufficient numbers to build up in the bowel.

Fortunately, pathogenic (harmful) bacteria represent less than two per cent of all species, and to cause disease there needs to be two important circumstances, namely:

1. a lowering of body resistance; and
2. contact with the harmful bacteria and/or their toxins.

Our bodies operate a number of defensive systems starting with the unbroken skin, which is a complete barrier to bacteria. If the skin is grazed or cut then white blood cells attack the invading bacteria. If that fails then the lymph glands act as filters, so causing the familiar swelling when infection is present. If the bacteria get past the glands into the blood stream, they can be attacked by white blood cells in the blood vessels, liver or spleen. The mucous membrane linings to most organs also attack bacteria as do substances known as antibodies which are formed in the body to resist a particular disease organism by natural or artifical immunisation. One of the most difficult control problems concerns the healthy carriers who are infected, recover often after a mild illness, but are not free of the bacteria. Thereafter such people may unknowingly continue to contaminate articles and food which subsequently can cause illness in other people.

There are four major groups of organisms responsible for bacterial food poisoning in Britain: *Salmonellae, Staphylococci, Clostridia* and *Bacillus cereus*.

Salmonella

Salmonella organisms are intestinal bacteria found in humans, animals and birds and are widely distributed throughout the world. To date over seventeen hundred different types have been identified. The following table gives an indication of the more common types of *Salmonellae* known to cause food poisoning, together with their common hosts.

TABLE 1

Salmonella Types	Host
S. typhi-murium	Rats, mice, dogs, cats, birds, ducks, hens and their eggs, calves, pigs
S. enteritidis	Cows, calves, pigs, turkeys, ducks, rats, mice, hens and their eggs
S. panama	Poultry, pigs, feeding stuffs, seafood
S. agona	Poultry, eggs, pigs, feeding stuffs
S. heidelberg	Poultry, eggs, pigs
S. virchow	Poultry, eggs, pigs, feeding stuffs
S. saint paul	Poultry, eggs, pigs, feeding stuffs
S. indiana	Poultry, pigs, feeding stuffs

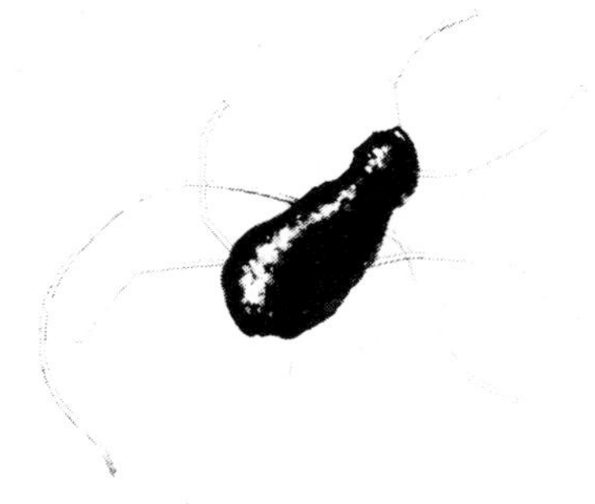

Salmonella typhimurium

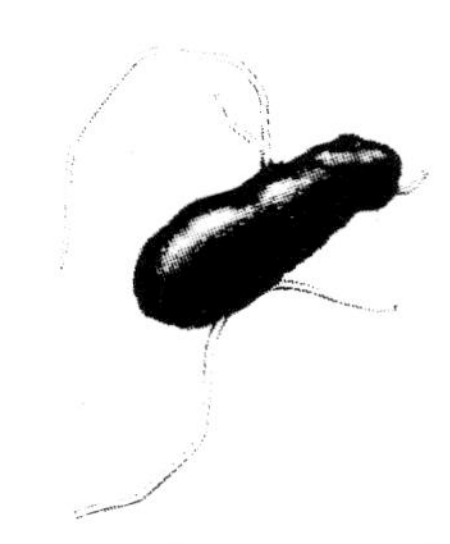

Salmonella enteritidis

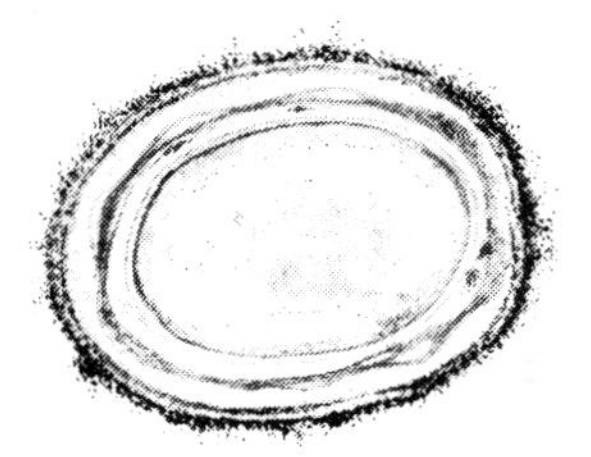

Clostridium botulinum type A

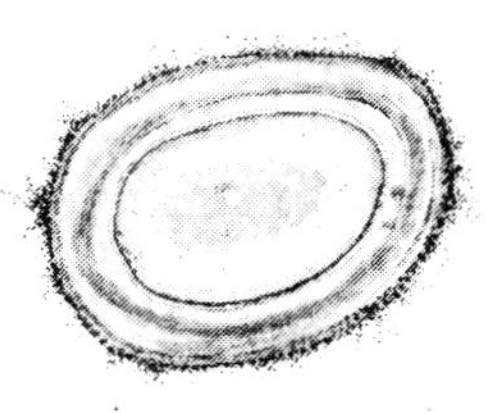

Clostridium perfringens (welchii) type C

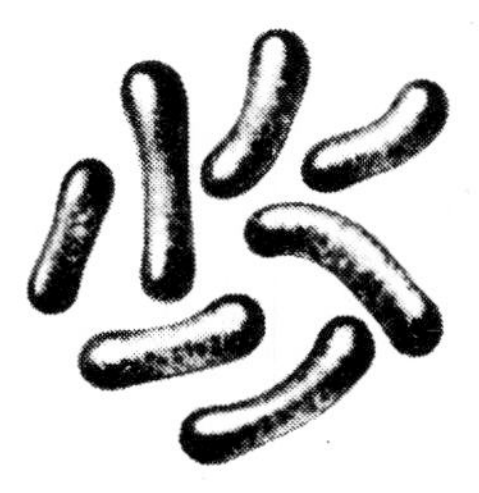

Bacillus cereus

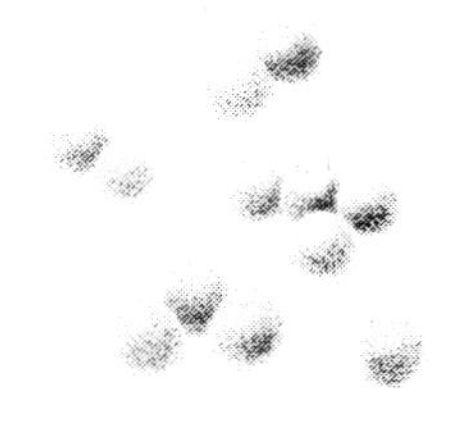

Staphylococcus aureus

Artist's impression — drawings not to the same scale. (By permission of Lever Industrial Ltd)

TABLE 2

Species of food animal	Census (millions)	Number Examined	% Positive S. typhi-murium	Estimated number positive of total population in Great Britain
Chickens	65.5	750	0.7	410,000
Pigs	2.2	600	7.0	154,000
Cattle	8.0	750	1.0	80,000
Ducks	0.8	650	2.5	20,000
Turkeys	2.2	500	1.2	26,000
Geese	0.8	100	2.0	16,000
Sheep	12.5	500	0.0	0

The figure in Table 2 were obtained from a national survey undertaken in 1969 and clearly show which meat animals and birds are potentially dangerous carriers of *Salmonella.* Subsequent surveys of fresh and frozen poultry have indicated a much higher incidence of infection — as high as 35 per cent being reported. It follows that many meat-based products are also potentially dangerous, although largely as a result of cross-contamination between raw and cooked meats. Canned meats are resonably safe because efficient processing at high temperatures destroys *Salmonellae;* reinfection after the can is opened is normally the source of the trouble.

Pasteurised milk is safe, but untreated milk is still sold and this product has been the cause of a number of outbreaks of *Salmonella* food poisoning in this country. The sale of untreated milk will be banned from 1 January 1980 in England and Wales.

Duck's eggs are almost invariably contaminated with *Salmonella* and this is one of the main reasons for giving them an extended period of boiling before consumption. Hen's eggs are less likely to be infected but imported eggs have a higher incidence rate and for some years regulations have prohibited the importation of frozen or powdered egg unless it has been subjected to pasteurisation.

Staphylococci

It has been suggested that up to 50 per cent of all people carry *Staphylococcus aureus* in their noses, throats, ears and on their hands, so common is the bacteria. Outbreaks of food poisoning due to this organism are caused by poor hygienic practices which result in food being contaminated by people, for example, sneezing over it; allowing food to come into contact with uncovered septic cuts or boils; or from healthy carriers. The bacteria (exterotoxins) can resist temperatures of 121°C (250°F) for 10 minutes, so they are not easily killed.

Clostridium welchii [perfringens]

This particular species of bacteria is commonly found in human and animal faecal matter and is frequently present in low numbers in raw meat. The organism forms spores which may survive boiling for several hours. Outbreaks of *Clostridium perfringens* food poisoning are associated with meat which may or may not have been insufficiently cooked, and which are cooled slowly, stored at room temperature rather than in a refrigerator, and either eaten cold or inadequately reheated the following day. High standards of personal hygiene assist in minimising the chances of contamination. Prevention of this type of food poisoning depends entirely on the suppression of growth of the organisms in the meat after cooking. Meat should be thoroughly cooked, cooled rapidly and stored in a refrigerator. If reheating is essential, it must be done thoroughly.

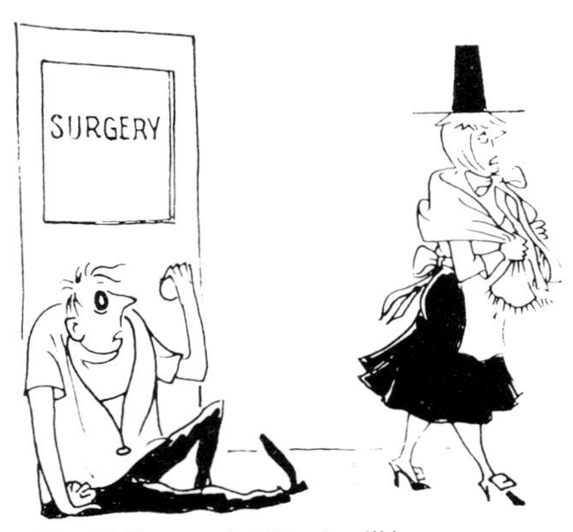

Clostridium welchii indeed"!

Bacillus cereus

This is a spore-forming bacterium commonly found in soil, on vegetation and in many raw and processed foods. In Britain many outbreaks of food poisoning caused by *B.cereus* have involved fried rice from Chinese restaurants. In these instances the incubation period varies, according to the quantity of infected food consumed, between thirty minutes and five hours. Symptoms include severe nausea and vomiting. The practice of boiling quantities of rice, subsequently allowing it to cool and remain at room temperature and then frying in beaten egg and oil appears to be the main cause of this form of food poisoning. Vanilla slices and ice cream have also been incriminated.

Vibrio parahaemolyticus

Vibrio parahaemolyticus is a common cause of food poisoning, principally from seafoods. The organism is found in shellfish, fish and sea water worldwide. Whilst raw food is naturally suspect, cooked seafood which has been contaminated during processing is equally dangerous. The incubation period for the disease varies from six to twenty hours.

Campylobacter

These bacteria have been known to cause several diseases in animals but until recently were not associated with human illness. Since 1974 the organism has been identified as the cause of acute enteritis (headache, nausea, diarrhoea and severe abdominal pain) in a number of patients. Evidence indicates that infected chickens, both live and dressed, are the primary source of the infection. The incubation period varies from two to eleven days and the illness lasts from a few days to three weeks.

From Table 3 it will be seen that food poisoning can be fatal, especially in the young and the elderly. The symptoms are very unpleasant in most instances; severe vomiting and stomach pains are frequently experienced and are commonly mistaken for appendicitis or even heart attacks. Diarrhoea and headaches are almost always a feature of the illness.

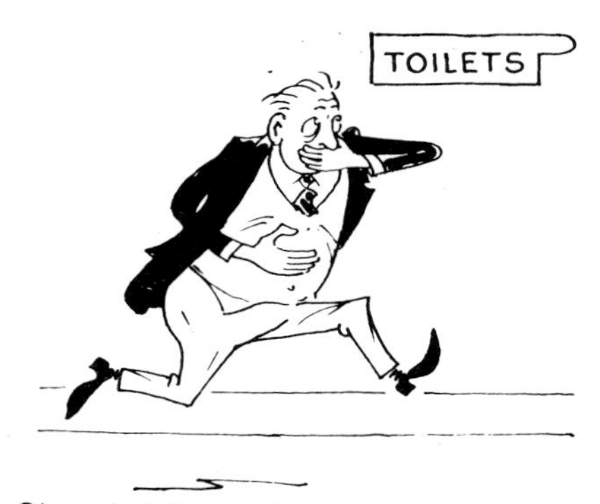

Characteristic symptoms

TABLE 3

Organism	Average Incubation Period	Symptoms	Average Recovery Period	Mortality Rate
Salmonella	8-24 hours Usually 18-24 hours	Nausea (with or without headache), abdominal pain, vomiting, diarrhoea, fever	2 days, but may last several weeks	Low 1.0%
Staphylococcus aureus	½-5 hours	Nausea, frequent vomiting, abdominal pain, persistent diarrhoea, prostration	Rapid, usually 5 hours after onset	Low 0.2%
Cl. Welchii	12 hours up to 18 hours	Diarrhoea, vomiting and abdominal cramp	2 days	Low
B. cereus Typical U.K. outbreaks	½-5 hours	Nausea and vomiting	1-2 days	Nil

Foods commonly associated with food poisoning

Readers will have already observed the classes of food identified with the various types of bacteria, and it will probably suffice to list the most common "danger" foods under broad headings.

TABLE 4

Meat and Meat Products	Dairy Products	Other foods
Beef	Milk	Fish
Veal	Cream	Crabs
Pork	Artificial cream	Oysters
Mutton	Cream cakes	Prawns and
Chicken	Custard	Other shellfish
Duck	Cheese	Rice
Turkey	Eggs	
Goose	Meringue	
Rabbit		
Meat Pies		
Ham & boiled bacon		
Sausages		
Canned meats		
Cooked meats		
Brawn		
Pâté		
Gravy and stock		

Methods of preservation

One age-old method of prolonging the shelf life of food has been the preservation of a variety of foods by drying. This originated with natural drying in the sun which removed the moisture which was vital to the growth of bacteria. This has developed into the accelerated freeze drying of food today.

Preservation by curing in salt has a long history, and also smoking to dry out the flesh. Sugar is another substance which bacteria dislike and which is used successfully as a preservative. In more recent times chemicals such as sulphur dioxide, benzoic acid and sodium nitrite and gases such as carbon dioxide have been used to store or preserve fruit in particular. Radiation sterilisation using ultra violet rays is also in use for some foods. Even antibiotics are being used in poultry, fish and cheese to prevent spoilage.

Canning was developed as a convenient packaging and preserving method during the nineteenth century and remains a popular and important part of the food industry. It should be realised that "sterile" products have received sufficient heat treatment to destroy *Cl. botulinum* and most spoilage organisms and that not all canned foods are commercially sterile and may need refrigeration:- e.g. large hams. Faulty canning can still, however, result in spoilage and waste.

Finally there has been the enormous growth in the use of freezing techniques to preserve a wide variety of foodstuffs. One important factor which must not be overlooked in this last method is that freezing does not always kill bacteria but merely suspends growth and reproduction until thawing occurs.

An all too common occurrence is food poisoning which has resulted from frozen poultry not being thawed properly prior to cooking. If the poultry is contaminated, unless it is thoroughly thawed, it will have the effect of countering the heat so that whilst the outer meat is cooked, the inner meat will not be subjected to a sufficiently high temperature to kill any bacteria present.

Food poisoning during processing

Other chapters will deal in detail with the techniques of food handling and cleansing of equipment, but the links between bacterial food poisoning and food processing are so fundamental that some reference should be made to the subject in this section.

One of the basic links in the chain of infection is the food handler, whether as a result of being a carrier, either knowingly or unknowingly, or as an intermediary responsible for transferring bacteria from one food or surface to another. One of the golden rules of catering is to avoid handling food more than absolutely necessary. Of equal importance is to observe strict personal hygiene, particularly keeping the hands scrupulously clean at all times, and not indulging in bad habits such as nose-picking, scratching and smoking. Clearly the state of the premises and the equipment play a part in good hygiene, so there is no substitute for the highest standards of cleanliness prevailing at all times. Above all, there is no doubt that safe practices and methods of food handling play a major part in preventing or avoiding outbreaks of food poisoning.

Reference has already been made to the large numbers of foods which can be potentially dangerous if allowed to be contaiminated by bacteria. Basically *food should be safely stored at the correct temperature* and then *carefully prepared* for sale or for consumption, *thoroughly cooked* and *served immediately.* Ideally food should not be kept hot for more than one hour, and during that time a temperature of over 82°C (150°F) should be maintained.

TABLE 5

Conditions contributing to 493 outbreaks of disease caused by foods processed in homes or in food service establishments.

Factor	No. of outbreaks
Inadequate refrigeration	336
Preparing food far in advance of service	156
Infected persons and poor personal hygiene	151
Inadequate cooking or heating	140
Holding food in warming device at too low a temperature	114
Contaminated raw materials in uncooked foods	84
Inadequate reheating	66
Cross-contamination	58
Inadequate cleaning of equipment	52
Other conditions	160

Other types of food poisoning

Apart from bacteria, food poisoning can be caused by animal, vegetable and chemical contamination.

Illness can result from the consumption of meat, fish and shellfish infected with the cystic stage of one of several parasites. Pork containing the cysts of *Trichinella spiralis* is responsible for Trichinosis, which is a painful disease affecting the eyes and face. Thorough cooking of food will kill any such cysts.

A number of exotic fish notably from Japan, such as "puffer fish" have occasionally been imported into this country and resulted in poisoning outbreaks, while the consumption of the roe of pike, sturgeon, carp, bream and turbot in the breeding season has also caused violent poisoning.

Vegetable poisoning is primarily due to the consumption of a poisonous fungus which is mistaken for a mushroom. This frequently results in death, especially if the death cap fungus is involved. Certain moulds can also produce lethal toxins — therefore avoid mouldy foods!

Poisonous weeds such as hemlock and monkshood have been mistaken for parsley and horseradish, while every country child is warned not to mistake deadly nightshade berries for cherries or redcurrants. The presence of oxalic acid in rhubarb leaves when used as a vegetable can lead to poisoning. Even potatoes have been the cause of illness due to the presence of excess solanine in the skin of baked potatoes.

Chemical poisoning is usually attributable to metallic concentrations of food following prolonged storage in cadmium, lead or copper pipes or containers. This is a particular problem with acid foods such as fruit, tomatoes and vinegar-based products. Consumption of contaminated food is likely to result in severe vomiting within two minutes to two hours. Food which has been contaminated with pesticides might also give rise to food poisoning type symptoms if eaten.

Some people are known to be allergic to certain food such as plums, strawberries, oysters or eggs; consumption of these will cause food poisoning type symptoms of sickness, nausea and headache, often accompanied by a skin rash. Once the sensitive food has been identified the only precaution is to avoid eating it.

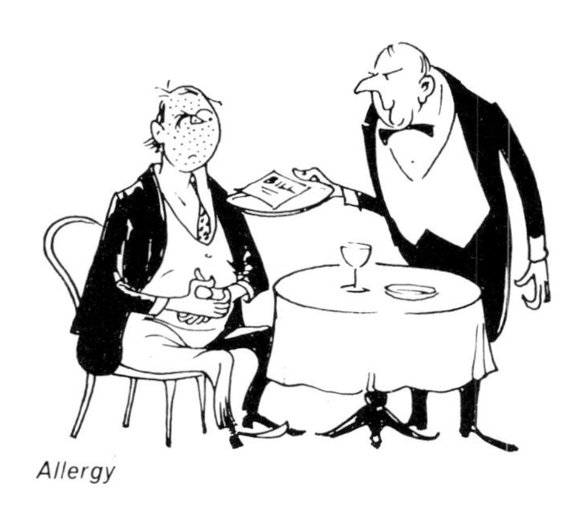

Allergy

Legal responsibilities

Food poisoning is a notifiable infectious disease, which means that a doctor is required by law (The Public Health Infectious Diseases Regulations, 1968) to notify the local authority of any case with which he is dealing. Many people who suffer from mild symptoms of food poisoning, such as diarrhoea, put it down to "having eaten too much fruit", or recover sufficiently not to trouble the hard-pressed doctor, and so many cases of food poisoning go unreported and undetected every day.

Unfortunately there is no easy diagnosis of food poisoning and the only method of identifying the offending bacteria is to take a faecal specimen from the sufferer and samples of suspected foodstuffs for examination in the laboratory. The examination is an involved and highly technical laboratory investigation which can take several days and even weeks if a particular *Salmonella* has to be identified from the 1700 different types. When the species of bacteria has been identified it is possible to subject the strain to further tests which will indicate which drugs will destroy the bacteria and which will be ineffective. This information is then reported to the doctor to enable a suitable course of treatment to be prescribed. Once the treatment is over, further faecal specimens will be necessary in order to ensure that the treatment was effective. In the case of *Salmonella* infections the incidence of cross-resistance effectively precludes any effective anti-biotic treatment.

Occasionally doctors fail to arrange for the necessary laboratory examination and prescribe a drug which may be ineffectual or even produce an immunity in the bacteria. This may result in the person becoming a "healthy carrier" for lengthy periods of time. It is probable that persons not troubling the doctor will also become healthy carriers who can remain undetected for months, possibly years in the case of typhoid carriers. If these carriers are also food handlers who are not careful of their personal hygiene, there is a very real risk that the bacteria will be spread via food to other people.

When a general practitioner notifies the local authority, the sufferer will usually receive a visit from an Environmental Health Officer who will not only arrange for the submisssion of faecal specimens before and after treatment, if prescribed, but will also investigate the likely cause of the food poisoning. Skilful detective work will often lead to an offending food or food premises and ultimately to the elimination of any further risk of food poisoning to the public at large. If the sufferer is a person engaged in the food trade the local authority has the legal power to prevent that person resuming work until satisfied that the person is free from infection. This procedure may involve the individual in several weeks' absence and in such cases the person may claim compensation for loss of earnings during the period of time.

The law also prohibits any person from working in a food business when suffering from any infectious disease or a bowel disorder, skin infection, nose or throat infection, and requires the person and/or proprietor to notify the local authority of any such occurrence.

In addition to requiring up to three negative faecal specimens before allowing a food handler to resume work after illness, many companies now require staff to submit routine faecal specimens for examination. The purpose of these checks is to identify carriers of food poisoning or gastro-enteritis bacteria, especially following a holiday abroad or an unspecified bout of illness. At least one large medical company offers a service to the food industry in which the staff are screened for *Salmonella* organisms and the results are notified to the company's medical adviser or the employee's general practitioner.

Finally, if an outbreak of food poisoning should occur in premises under your control, the following action should be taken.

1. Telephone the local Evironmental Health Department (unless they bring the bad news). Outside normal office hours there is usually an emergency number in the telephone directory.
2. If customers are ill on the premises, call an ambulance or local doctor.
3. If possible keep any food similar to that eaten by them.
4. Do not throw anything away or start cleaning until advised to do so.
5. Make a list of the staff on duty and the names and addresses of any staff off duty, together with the reason for their absence.
6. Prepare a list of your food suppliers:- e.g., butcher, wholesale grocer, baker.
7. Prepare a set of menu cards for the past 48 hours. Ideally a sample dish from each type of meal served in the previous 48 hours should be available for examination.

This information and assistance will be invaluable to the Environmental Health Officer in his efforts to identify the cause of the outbreak and to advise on ways of preventing a recurrence.

Some Case Histories

The following case histories will give readers some idea of the scale of food poisoning outbreaks occurring in Britain.

(1) At 10.30 a.m., a husband and wife on a day trip consumed sandwiches made two hours earlier by the wife from a freshly-opened 7 oz can of chopped pork. The unused part of the meat was placed in a sealed container in a refrigerator and the tin put in a waste bin. At 12.30 p.m., the husband was violently sick and collapsed. At 3 p.m., his wife became violently sick and also collapsed. Examination of the unused pork and the discarded tin revealed *Staphylococcus aureus* which was also isolated from the faeces of the two patients. Examination of the tin and other tins from the same batch obtained from the shop indicated that the seaming at both ends of the can was completely inadequate. Further imports of products from the factory in question were banned until canning techniques were improved.

(2) Within thirty-six to forty-eight hours of their arrival on a Saturday at the same hotel, forty-two of the seventy-one guests, members

of two separate coach parties from different parts of the country, became ill. Most of them had diarrhoea, vomiting and abdominal cramp; four had diarrhoea only and four vomiting only. Faecal specimens were submitted for examination by 34 patients, and *C. welchii* were isolated from seven. No other pathogens were isolated.

Before the onset of illness, the guests had eaten three meals (excluding breakfast) at the hotel. On the first evening the meal included roast beef and gravy, lunch on Sunday was roast chicken with gravy, and the evening meal on Sunday was a ham salad. One of those feeling ill was a vegetarian who admitted to having eaten gravy on Saturday evening and at Sunday lunchtime. No food was available for bacteriological examination.

Faecal specimens from 15 kitchen staff were also submitted for examination and *C.welchii* were isolated from five of these. The staff had not suffered from diarrhoea.

The kitchen premises of the hotel and procedures for the preparation, cooking and storage of food, particularly meat and gravy, were being intensively investigated by the local Health Department.

(**3**) Three persons had vomiting and diarrhoea two to three hours after eating fried rice at a Chinese restaurant. *Bacillus cereus* was isolated from the rice but not from other food examined.

(**4**) Thirty out of sixty-three persons at a boarding school had diarrhoea ten hours after eating cold mutton. The meat was cooked the previous day and left in the oven overnight; it was reheated for lunch and then served cold for tea. *C.welchii* was isolated from ten persons examined and from the cold meat.

(**5**) Two persons had vomiting and diarrhoea four to six hours after eating cake. *Staphylococcus aureus* was isolated from the cake filling which consisted of crumbled sponge fingers, margarine, icing sugar and canned pear juice; it was kept at room temperature for two days. *Staphylococcus aureus* was also isolated from a food handler (ear, nose and skin swabs).

(**6**) On 10 January, 280 staff members of a factory in the Calderdale area ate a buffet supper. 80 are known to have become ill with diarrhoea and abdominal pain after about two to three days; fifty-six were positive for *Salmonella hadar*.

Although a number of cold meats had been consumed, the only remnants available were parts of one of three 13 kg (28 lb) frozen turkeys. These had been given to an old lady who had passed some on to another family, all of whom had diarrhoea. These remnants, examined after several days, contained *S.hadar*.

The turkeys were supplied by a producer/slaughterer who killed them on 19 December, removed them from the freezer on 5 January, and delivered them on 7 January. They were kept at room temperature and then cooked separately, in three batches, in a small domestic oven on 8 and 9 January. The exact times and temperature of cooking were not known, and inconsistent stories were given. They were then kept at room temperature in an unventilated kitchen until sliced and served on 10 January. Defrosting appears to have been adequate, but there is some doubt about the adequacy of cooking, because the meat was still pink near the bone, and there is no doubt that the birds were kept for thirty-six to forty-eight hours at warm room temperature after being cooked.

(7) Between October and November, eleven clinical cases of salmonellosis, due to the organism, occurred in one small area, together with two isolations from symptomless individuals.

Investigation of possible food sources was prolonged but six of the eleven cases had eaten pork pies produced at one small factory and another case worked in the butcher's shop attached to it. There was a clear geographical relationship of cases to butcher' shops which sold these particular pies. The organism was found in one pork pie from the factory.

Faecal samples from four food-handling workers were examined and *S.kapemba* was discovered in one man who admitted to having an intestinal illness in September which he had not reported. He normally handled only raw meat but occasionally added the jelly to the cooked pies. As the mechanical jellying machine was broken he used his unprotected forefinger to pierce the cooked pies and then poured in the jelly. Following his removal from work, no further isolations have been made.

(Public Health Laboratory Service — unpublished reports)

Chapter 3

DESIGN AND CONSTRUCTION OF FOOD PREMISES

The difficulty in considering the design and construction of any food premises is that so much depends on the type and volume of the anticipated business. As so often happens, this volume of business is under-estimated to the extent that the premises become too small with the almost inevitable result that problems arise in connection with the storage, preparation and production of food.

In designing new premises, an accurate assessment of likely trade is essential for a proper balance to be made in the allocation of space. There is no point in planning a restaurant with seating for 200 customers, if the kitchen is only suitable for preparing fifty meals at any one time.

Equally there is little point in planning a shop where the anticipated retail trade far exceeds the back-up storage capacity. The economic viability of the business must be carefully calculated beforehand, in the knowledge that a food business means far more than just "selling".

Perhaps most problems are experienced where existing premises, which were never originally designed as food premises, have to be adapted; although careful planning and the sensible use of materials and equipment can help to make the best use of limited space. Certainly the careful design and choice of equipment in any food premises will not only make good hygiene an easier process, but also will encourage clean habits in the staff.

The basic lay-out and construction should be designed to enable:

1. Adequate space to be provided in all food handling and associated areas; and
2. Frequent and routine cleaning to be carried out.

Food preparation rooms should be planned to allow a "work flow", whereby food is processed through the premises from the point of delivery to the point of sale or service with the minimum obstruction. The various processes should be separated as far as possible and food intended for sale should not cross paths with waste food or refuse. Staff time is valuable and

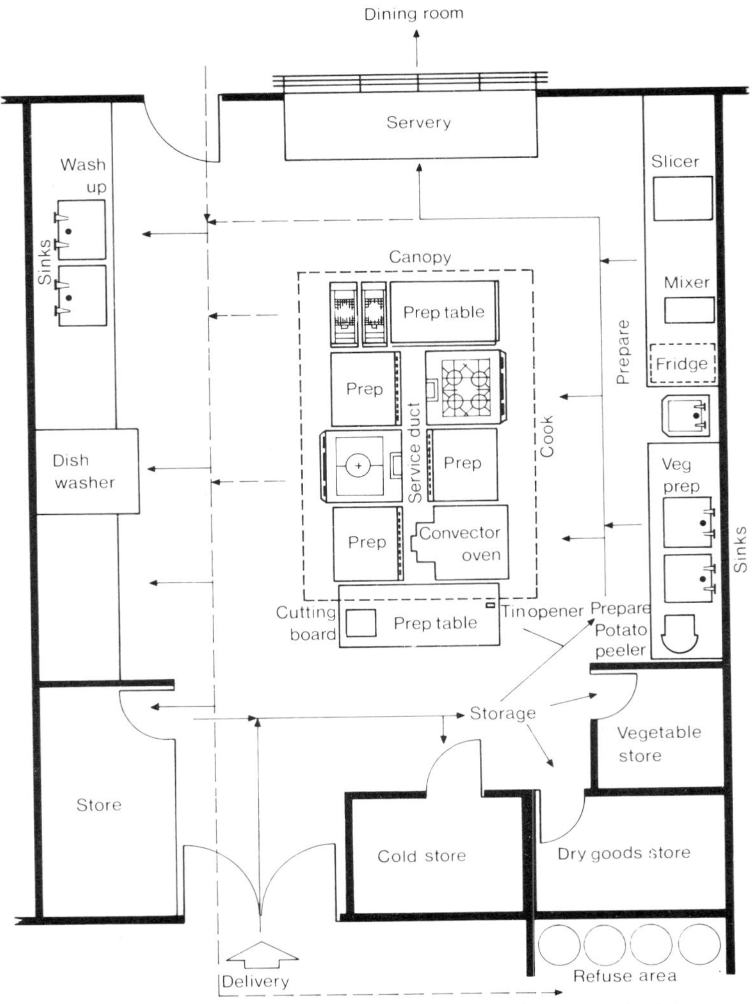

"Work Flow" diagram showing optimum use of space and minimum interference from other workers

a design which reduces wasteful journeys is both efficient and cost effective.

The various preparation processes require different types of consideration depending on what food is involved. A vegetable preparation area means that water from the sinks and dirt from the vegetables are going to accumulate and therefore adequate facilities for drainage should be provided. Pastry preparation, on the other hand, entails dry processes, although flour is likely to be released into the atmosphere which can create problems with cleaning.

Whatever the process, however, there are certain basic rules that can be applied which not only make for easier working conditions but which also help in making the requirements of the Food Hygiene Regulations a reality.

Given that one has an existing shell of a building, care should be taken in the very first instance to see that, before specific areas are allocated, adequate space is provided for the preparation of food, storage, sales and service, staff facilities and the storage of refuse.

The various methods of storing food are dealt with in Chapter 6, but it will suffice to say at this stage that foodstuffs should not be stored in passageways or in food preparation areas where they will not only impede staff working there but also will hamper proper cleaning.

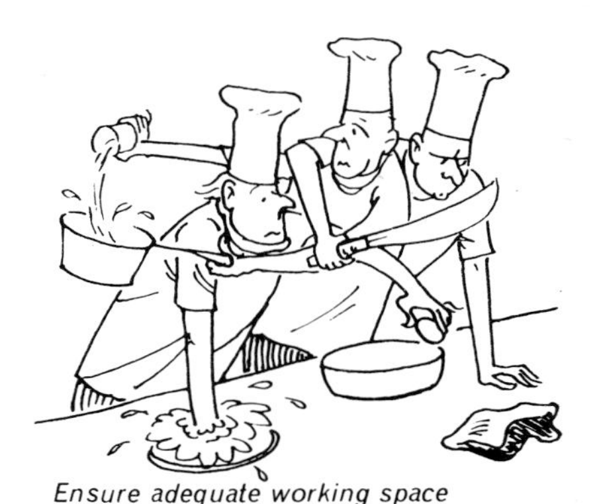

Ensure adequate working space

Food Preparation Areas

There is no doubt that the proper design and lay-out of the preparation area can make a major contribution to good food hygiene. It is also true that staff generally respond to good working conditions by taking more of a pride in themselves and in what they are doing.

Adequate space must be provided for each process and care should be taken to separate dirty and clean areas. Vegetable preparation and wash-up areas should be separate from the actual food preparation or service areas. As with the lay-out of premises, a work flow arrangement should be introduced so that staff do not hamper each other by having to cross each other's paths more than is absolutely necessary.

Actual work-top areas should be adequate in size for the preparation process and should enable the food handler to have all the necessary food and utensils near to hand. Stainless steel (18/8 quality) is an ideal material for use in catering premises for work-tops and in the construction of most pieces of equipment. An inferior alternative is a plastic laminate veneer finish, although this is far preferable to wood in any situation. Wood tends to be absorbent and easily damaged, with consequent cleaning difficulties.

Floors

The basic rule is that these should be smooth, impervious (water and grease proof), and capable of being readily cleaned. At the same time they should not be slippery or in any other way dangerous. Floors should generally be solid, whilst the choice of finish will usually depend on the type of food business. In a kitchen, quarry tiles, granolithic or terrazzo are best because they are hard-wearing, will withstand grease and water and can be easily cleaned. Floors in storerooms or retail areas may be similarly surfaced, although industrial sheet linoleum or vinyl may be acceptable where there are dry conditions, and provided a suitable adhesive is used. Wooden floors are not acceptable as a general rule because, even if they have been sealed, dirt may collect in cracks and joints. An additional hazard, where there are wooden suspended floors, is the risk of harbourage for rodents and insects. Concrete floors are not suitable in most food rooms because the surface can break down and cause dust. Although the surface can be sealed, concrete should not be used where there is likely to be heavy wear.

Where quantities of water are likely to find their way on to the floor, or in an area where wet cleaning is the best way of removing deposits, adequate drainage should be provided, either by a central gully to which the floor is sloped or by a channel situated along one of the walls — to which again the floor is inclined. Grids and grease traps should be provided to filter out material that might obstruct the draining system and full access should be provided to permit proper cleaning. The use of newspaper, cardboard, sawdust or carpet on floors is not acceptable. The installation of non-slip floor tiles is recommended wherever slippery conditions are encountered.

Walls

Again the general rule of being smooth, impervious and capable of being readily cleaned should be applied. The walls themselves should be surfaced to prevent any intervening gap in which insects or rodents might be harboured. Where possible, walls should be coved with the floor to enable easy cleaning.

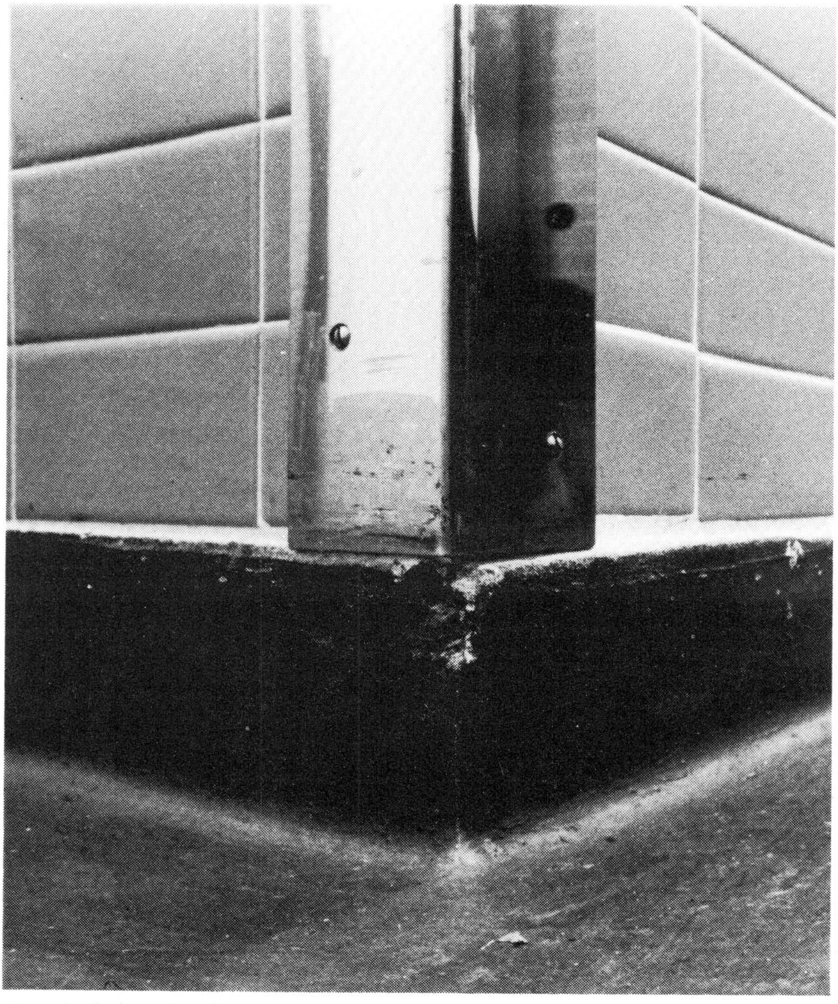

A typical example of wall to floor coving

Glazed tiles or stainless steel sheets provide the most suitable surfaces for food rooms, although the former should not be used near to sources of heat such as cookers, otherwise they will crack. In kitchens and other food preparation areas, the most vulnerable areas are those up to approximately 1.5 metres (5ft) and it may be sufficient merely to tile to that height. Wall areas where there are likely to be special problems, for example, near cookers or where they are likely to be knocked, should be covered with stainless steel or similar sheeting. Tiles should be laid evenly on a sound base and the jointing compound should be mixed with gloss paint as a sealer to prevent absorption. Other areas may be covered with laminated sheeting or gloss painted, but care should be taken with the sheeting to ensure that no voids are created behind.

The choice of tiles and paint is important not only from an aesthetic point of view, but also with regard to safe working conditions. Light colours show up dirt better, besides which they make the best use of available light. The use of metal edging strips around doorways is a sensible precaution against accidental damage by trolleys, etc.

Walls should be as clear of obstruction as possible to enable easy cleaning. The pinning or taping up of posters or notices should be discouraged.

Wall surfaces in retail shops may not need the attention required in a kitchen, although again smooth and impervious finishers are essential. The use of gloss paint may, however, be extended, particularly where the walls are unlikely to be exposed to either damage or extremes of temperature.

Wallpaper should not be used in food preparation rooms, although there are some washable varieties which may sometimes be used in dry areas such as in retail shops.

Pipework, ducting and so on should be chased into the wall or floor, or constructed tight to the ceiling to enable an effective seal to be made. Horizontal pipework collects dust and dirt and frequently results in condensation. This causes dripping which can contaminate any uncovered food beneath.

Ceilings

The choice of materials for ceilings presents particular problems because they may be exposed to extremes of temperature, fumes and steam, and are not readily accessible for cleaning. Ceilings should be capable of being easily cleaned by being smooth, but should also be partially absorbent. Otherwise, in moist conditions, condensation will arise which may result in droplets falling on to food, thus causing contamination.

The most suitable material is plasterboard sheeting, where the joints are taped and a skim coat of plaster applied to prevent harbourage of dirt. This type of surface is slightly absorbent, yet can be wiped over to remove heavy concentrations of dirt. It also has the advantage of being able to be emulsioned when it becomes discoloured.

Gloss finishes should be avoided and, where possible, fibreglass insulation should be provided behind the main surface. This will help to reduce the risk of condensation.

The height of the ceiling will often have a bearing on the conditions in the food room and particularly in a kitchen. If the ceiling is too high, it can create cold working conditions and means that the ceiling is less accessible for cleaning. On the other hand, without adequate ventilation, a low ceiling may create temperatures that are too high for comfortable working. Much will depend on the extent of the food preparation but, in an average size kitchen, a ceiling of approximately 3-3.6 metres (10-12 ft) will not only ensure that the ceiling is accessible for cleaning but will also mean that extremes of temperature are unlikely to arise.

As with wall surfaces, care should be taken to avoid a suspended ceiling, which may create a breeding ground for insects or rodents.

Doors, Windows and Stairs

Many parts of the food premises must, of necessity, be made of wood. Where this is so, they should be designed to prevent the accumulation of dirt and to facilitate easy cleaning. Doors should be of plain rather than patterned construction and window frames should be simple rather than complicated.

Doors should generally have finger plates to facilitate easy cleaning where hands are most likely to come into contact. A metal plate fixed to the bottom 15-20 cm (6-9 in) and metal edging strips around the sides of the door will prevent damage by people kicking it open, and by trolleys, etc. On outside doors it acts as a deterrent to gnawing rodents.

Catches, handles and other door and window fittings should be made of aluminium, which is rust-proof, does not need painting and which is obtainable in various, easy-to-clean designs. Many industrial food premises have installed polypropylene or toughened rubber doors incorporating self-closing devices. These have advantages from a food hygiene standpoint and they may also be required in connection with fire prevention.

Stairs should be designed to provide a straight access between floors with an adequate width, easy pitch (not too steep) and handrails for safety.

Good natural and artificial lighting is essential and special attention should be paid to the construction and surfacing of stairs. A non-slip tread should be provided wherever possible. Carpeting should be avoided because of the cleaning and maintenance problems.

Ventilation

Ventilation is a process which provides an adequate supply of clean, fresh air, generally from the outside. It is basically dependent upon a movement or circulation of air at a sufficient rate to ensure that moist, stale air is removed at regular intervals.

Adequate ventilation is essential in any kitchen, not only for the welfare of the staff, but also because high temperatures are going to promote the growth of bacteria on the more vulnerable foods. Inadequate ventilation will also contribute to the cleaning bill because, if grease and steam-laden fumes are allowed to remain in the kitchen, they will condense on to surfaces making effective cleaning much more difficult.

Ventilation can be achieved either naturally or artificially. Natural ventilation can be supplied through windows and doors although clearly, in cold weather, it may not always be convenient to have all the necessary windows open. Open windows also have the added disadvantage of admitting dust and insects, although the latter can be controlled by fitting perforated gauze coverings. Any covering will, however, restrict the circulation of air, can be difficult to clean and may be easily broken. Although a kitchen may have sufficient windows, they may not be positioned to give the most effective circulation when open and their constant opening and closing by food handlers can present an additional hazard through hands touching fitments which have become contaminated. Most kitchens therefore will need some form of mechanical ventilation, especially those which are of peculiar shape, size, below ground level, or enclosed within a building.

The caterer will need expert advice on deciding which type of ventilation is best for his premises but, as a general rule in deciding on the design of the system, it is always better to overestimate than underestimate. Although the initial cost may be higher, the long-term advantages will justify the expense. There are many heating and ventilation engineers available for advice.

The simplest type of mechanical ventilation can be an electric extractor fan fitted into an external wall or window and operated by either a pull cord or switch. Pull cords, incidentally, are not recommended because of the difficulty in cleaning them. The positioning of the fan is important. It should be placed to pick up the majority of the fumes from the kitchen. Externally it should not be allowed to discharge at the face level of passers-by or where the discharge might carry to other rooms.

It has been suggested that one should aim at about 20 air changes per hour in a large kitchen. Although some say that this rate is too high, mechanical ventilation will still be necessary if one is to achieve 10 to 15 changes per hour.

Apart from creating a circulation and renewal of the total air within a room, one should pay individual attention to particular sources of heat, fume or steam. Cooking ranges, fryers and boilers all release large volumes of fumes into the atmosphere and special provision should be made to control this effluvia. The simplest way is to collect the fumes inside a hood which connects to a duct leading to the outside air. The ducting should incorporate a fan which will create an air current away from the source and a filter arrangement to arrest the majority of heavy material such as grease particles. The fan will normally be situated as far from the source of heat as possible to prevent damage to the motor, while the filter will be near to the source in order to absorb as much grease and dirt as possible and thereby prevent any build-up in the ducting.

In a large kitchen, the best position for the cooking range is in the centre. This permits easier access for cleaning around and underneath the equipment, and also it does give an opportunity to install a canopy arrangement overhead. Canopies come in a variety of shapes and sizes but, as a rule, they should be of stainless and rust-proof metal without hidden corners and voids in which dust can collect. They should not be so high that fumes can escape into the room or so low that staff can knock their heads on them. The filter, which may be of wire wool or similar material, should be readily accessible for easy removal and cleaning. Any fan housing should likewise be accessible.

Many modern buildings in this country are equipped with air conditioning which provides a balanced system of purified air into each part of the building, and a separate ducted extraction of stale air. The design should make special allowance for the catering activities.

Lighting

While premises should take the fullest advantage of natural lighting through large, well-placed windows, efficient artificial lighting is essential throughout the food premises for three main reasons:

1. to enable staff to work in an agreeable environment and to see what they are doing;

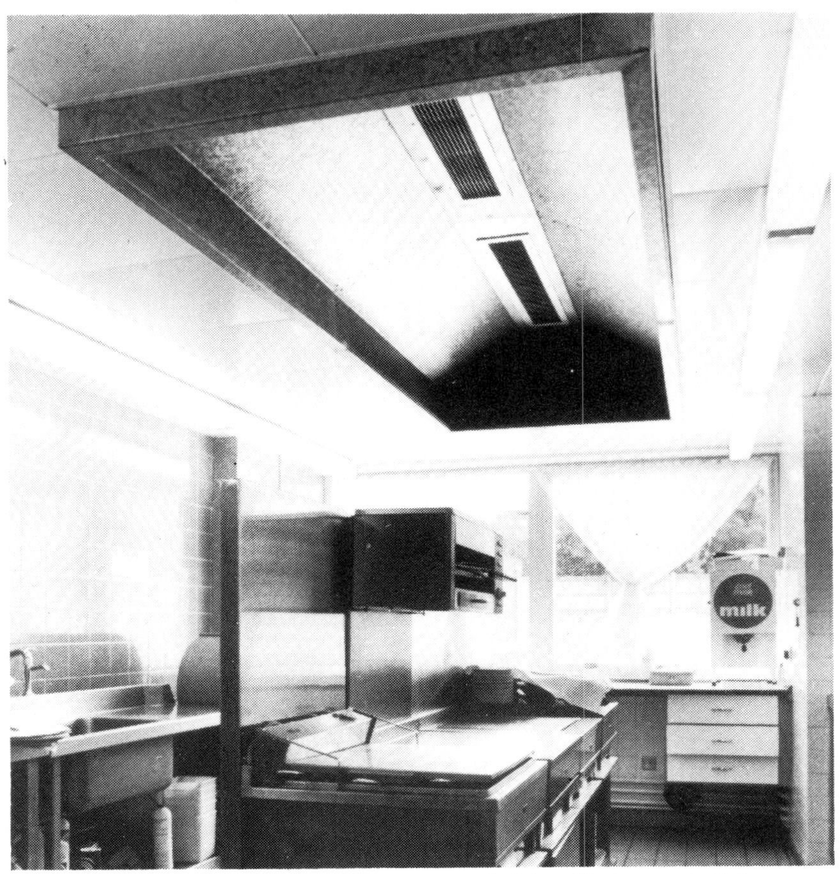

A well-designed ventilation hood over a central "island"; the area is lit by fluorescent strip lighting units

2. to facilitate adequate cleaning by revealing what might otherwise be "hidden spots"; and
3. to prevent accidents.

Adequate lighting should not be confined to the main work areas but should also be provided in passageways, store rooms, on stairs and in those areas outside a building where staff need to go, such as refuse areas or delivery bays. The design of premises can do much to procure adequate lighting by ensuring that areas are as open as possible, without unnecessary walls or other obstructions. Wall and ceiling finishes can be chosen to enhance available light by using light-reflecting colours.

The number and capacity of lights required in any particular place will obviously depend on the size of the area to be illuminated. From a working point of view, a number of independent lights, positioned over those areas where people work, are preferable to fewer large-wattage lights, which will need to be positioned fairly high to spread the light and which may well lose its intensity and cause shadows in the process. Glare from unshaded lights or working in inadequately-lit surroundings will cause fatigue and can damage the eyes. A level of 400 lux on working surfaces is recommended.

The choice of equipment is important. Fluorescent lights will give a more efficient light than the traditional bulb, besides it is easier for a tube to be covered with a shade which will disperse the light evenly. Both tubes and shades can be selected to give a light most agreeable to those working on the premises and without glare. Most designs are fairly easy to keep clean. Tubes also have a longer life and are cheaper to run than tungsten-filament bulbs.

All light fittings, including switches, should be of simple design and preferably flush with the ceiling or wall to permit easy cleaning. Press button switches or those with recesses should be avoided as it is easy for food deposits to build up on them.

Those electrical fittings which are situated near to sinks, cooking ranges or refrigerators should be sealed to keep out moisture and should preferably be of either rubber, plastic or rust-proof metal. Wiring should be laid in conduits and, where possible, chased into the wall to avoid unnecessary dust traps.

In a large kitchen it may be preferable to have individual lights, or groups of lights, operated by separate switches. This not only saves electricity and offers a greater flexibility, but also eliminates the need to have large clusters of switches which may become difficult to clean.

Some food rooms may conveniently be fitted with "illuminated ceilings". These consist of a series of fluorescent tubes situated behind a translucent screen. This has the advantage of dispersing the light efficiently, also the surface can be easily cleaned. The main disadvantage, however, is that dust and dirt may find its way behind the screen and create what can become a harbourage for insects.

Refuse Storage

Refuse containers must be situated outside the building, preferably in a covered, though not totally enclosed, area.

This is because any such area will be much more difficult to clean if the refuse is wet. However, if the area is roofed and semi-enclosed, this ensures that there is adequate ventilation.

Refuse can be divided into two types: dry waste, which includes paper, cardboard and boxes; and wet waste, which includes food and general kitchen debris.

The best type of container for wet waste is either a metal or plastic bin with a close-fitting lid which keeps out flies and other insects. The bins should be sited off the ground on racks to allow for easy cleaning and to make the lifting process less arduous.

Dry waste should also be stored off the ground and should, as far as possible, be compacted. This makes collection easier and ensures the maximum use of the available space. Where there are large quantities of paper and cardboard involved, a compaction unit can be installed which compresses the waste into manageable bales.

Where space is at a premium, and where there is no need to separate the refuse, it may be possible to install one of the many types of bulk containers that are marketed. These are of approximately 1 cubic metre (35 cubic ft) capacity and can replace up to 8 dustbins. The containers are fitted with wheels and, as they are lifted and emptied by a

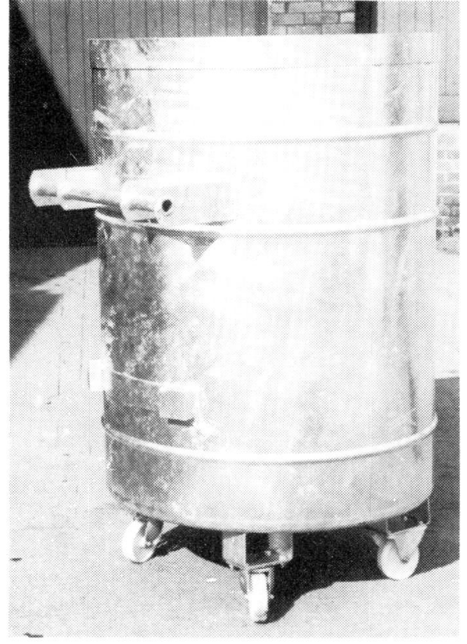

A bulk container (Trevor Iles & Co. Ltd)

specially-adapted vehicle, road access must be provided or it must be possible for the container itself to be wheeled to the vehicle. The local authority usually advise on the type of bulk container which fits their vehicles. Alternatively, many private waste-disposal firms operate very efficient services and provide their own containers.

Both dustbins and bulk containers need to be kept clean and should be regularly cleansed to prevent food accumulating which might attract flies or give rise to offensive smells. Many councils and private operators of bulk container systems include a steam-cleaning service and traders are well advised to pay the small extra charge for this. If flies or smells do present a problem, particularly in hot weather, various aerosols or dusting powders are available which should be applied regularly.

In all cases, refuse needs to be collected regularly by either the local authority or private contractors. The frequency will depend upon the volume of refuse generated by the business and could be daily.

The working waste generated in a kitchen during the day is best kept in either plastic bags or bins within the kitchen. These should be renewed or cleansed as necessary at the end of each working day. Waste food should never be stored within the food premises overnight.

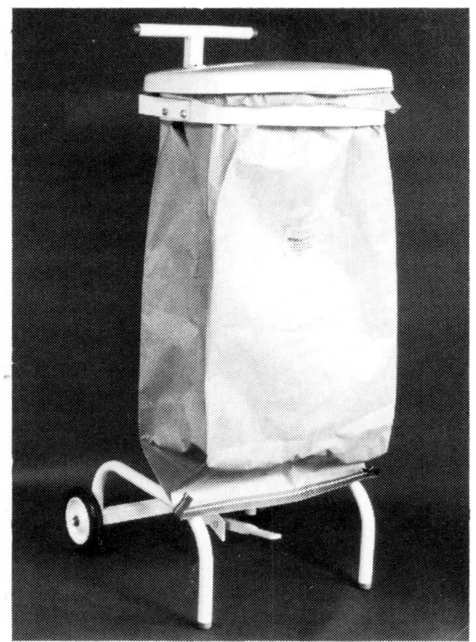

Refuse sack holder (Trevor Iles & Co. Ltd)

Most wet waste can be removed by using a disposal unit. These are fitted beneath the outlet of the sink and incorporate an electrical grinding mechanism, reducing the waste to small particles, which can then be sluiced to the drain.

The refuse area itself should have an impervious floor such as concrete, which is well drained to assist with washing down. Walls should be smooth and impervious for easy cleaning and the area generally should be well lighted, both naturally and artificially. The junction of the walls and floor should be coved to prevent the accumulation of waste.

Sanitary Conveniences and Staff Cloakrooms

All food premises should have adequate sanitary accommodation for staff and, where appropriate, separate accommodation for the public. The accommodation should be readily accessible to staff and while in smaller premises, where only one or two are employed, a single lavatory may suffice; in larger premises involving numbers of employees, it will be necessary to have separate accommodation for each sex, which should be situated at each floor level.

Sanitary conveniences must be kept clean and in efficient working order. They should be so constructed that the walls, floor and ceiling are finished with a smooth, impervious material which is capable of being readily cleaned. Every compartment should be adequately lighted and should be ventilated to the outside air. In the case of a compartment not having a window, effective ventilation can be achieved by using a system of ducts, incorporating an extractor fan worked in conjunction with the light switch, and an electrical overrun device to provide at least 3 air changes per hour.

Although lavatories must be conveniently situated within the food premises, they must not be directly entered from a food room, so as to avoid offensive odours penetrating into the latter. It is necessary to provide an intervening lobby between the food room and the sanitary convenience and this should be well ventilated. Neither the compartment containing the sanitary convenience nor the intervening lobby may be used for the storage of food.

It is a requirement of the law that there has to be displayed, in a conspicuous position near to the sanitary convenience, a legible notice clearly requesting users to wash their hands after using the convenience.

Although it may be necessary to provide suitable washhand basins elsewhere in the food premises, it is important that one or more basins be situated conveniently near to the sanitary conveniences so that staff may

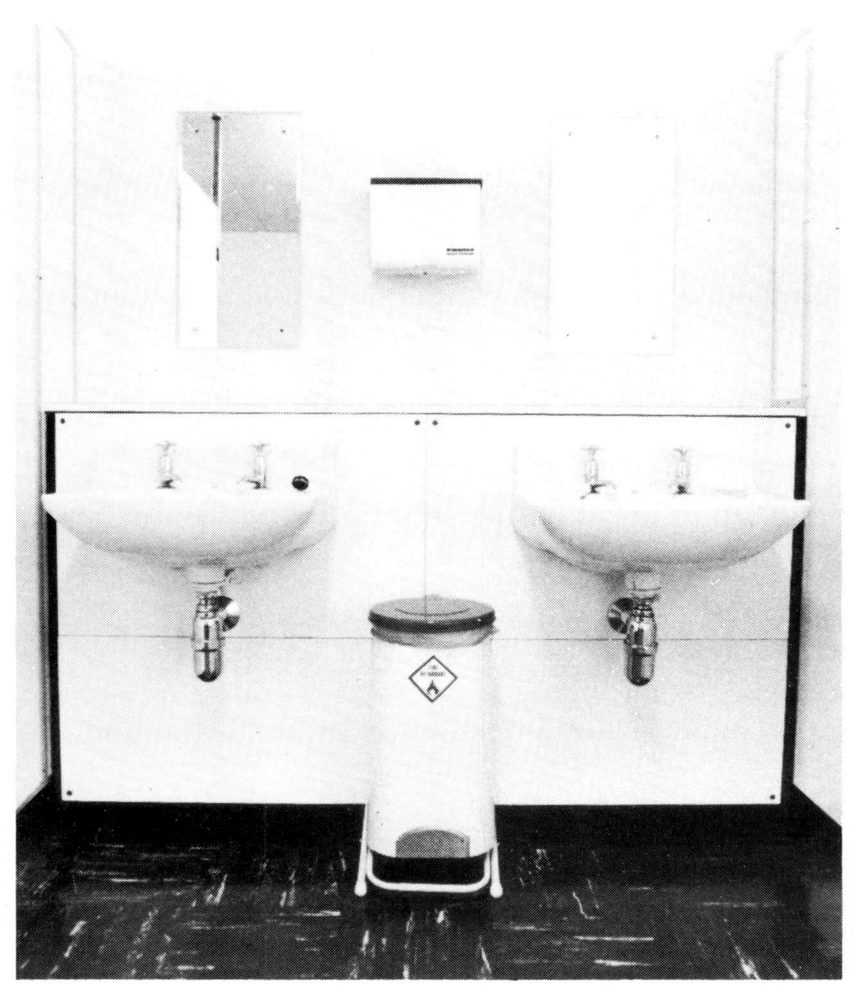

Well-designed staff washing facilities. Note the centrally placed paper towel dispenser and waste bin

wash their hands having used the lavatory. The wash basins can be situated within the intervening lobby and should be provided with hot and cold water supplies or with hot water at a suitable controlled temperature, soap or liquid detergent, a nail brush and suitable means for hand drying.

In the case of separate conveniences for the sexes, outermost doors should be conspicuously labelled as being for each sex and, in order to maintain an effective intervening space between the sanitary convenience and the food room, the doors should be self-closing.

Adequate accommodation for the outdoor or other clothing and footwear not worn by the staff during normal working hours, must be provided. These articles of clothing must not be stored in a food room and should be stored in separate lockers allocated to each member of staff. Although these lockers may be situated in a food room, it is recommended that a separate room be designated as a cloakroom so that clothes can be stored there conveniently. In the event of outdoor clothing becoming wet, they can be more readily dried than if contained within a small locker. Adequate washing facilities should be provided in the cloakroom, which will not only encourage staff to wash their hands before starting and after finishing their work, but will also act as a reminder that personal hygiene and washing is important. Cloakrooms should be properly maintained and the same general standards for the cleanliness of the food premises should apply.

Chapter 4

THE DESIGN OF EQUIPMENT

While the design and maintenance of food premises will be a major influence on whether food hygiene standards are good or bad, the choice of equipment will also influence standards to a very great extent. The condition of equipment must be viewed in two ways:

1. Is it clean?
2. Having regard to its physical condition — is it worn or broken?

Both of these criteria are important because any equipment is a potential danger if, by reason of its condition, it cannot be properly cleaned. It is a danger because dirt may accumulate in cracks, hidden corners or within the material with which the equipment has been constructed and that dirt may, in turn, harbour those bacteria which could give rise to food poisoning. Equally, given the very best equipment, unless it is kept clean there is always the danger of harmful bacteria being transferred to the food.

The Food Hygiene Regulations should influence the design, construction and subsequent maintenance of any equipment. The Regulations require equipment not only to be clean but also to be in such condition that it can be thoroughly cleaned. The Regulations go further by insisting that equipment shall not be absorbent and that it shall not present any risk of contamination to the food with which it comes into contact.

In effect, these criteria mean that equipment, with few exceptions, must be made from materials that are smooth, impervious and capable of being readily cleaned. This is a golden rule for the caterer and one that can be applied both to his choice of equipment and to the construction of his premises. Looking at equipment in the form of tables and other preparation areas first, it means that wood should not be used where open food is prepared or stored, the reason being that it simply cannot be adequately cleaned. All woods to a greater or lesser degree are absorbent. The softer woods, even when new, are absorbent and tests have shown that fluids can be "drawn" into the body of a wooden table top to a depth of several inches. This being the case, one can assume that bacteria can likewise be drawn into the body of the wood. Once there, normal superficial cleaning, though resulting in conditions appearing clean to the naked eye, will not remove or destroy them. The result is that those bacteria can then transfer to other food which is placed on the table.

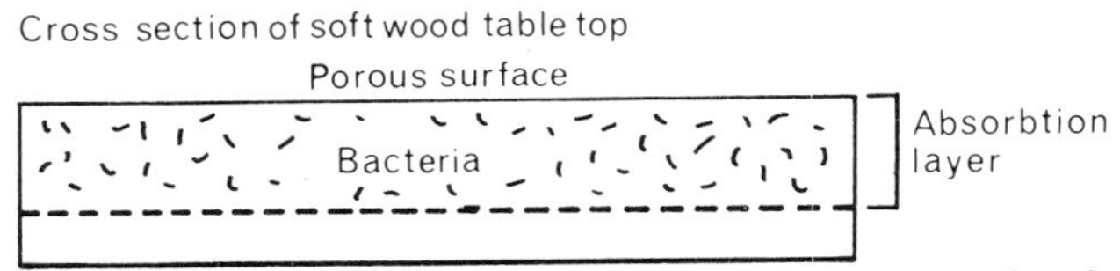

The vulnerability of wooden table tops to contamination

The aim, therefore, in any catering establishment must be to eliminate the use of soft wood whenever possible. This extends to the use of plastic-backed nail brushes and plastic broom handles instead of the traditional wooden ones.

The use of wood

There will be parts of equipment in the catering premises which may utilise wood in their construction. Wooden legs to tables, shelves in a dry store or duck boards on the floor may be used, although only as a second choice to stainless steel or similar metal. They should be sealed by using three coats of polyurethane varnish. The surface to be treated should first be cleaned of any visible dirt, then steeped in a disinfectant solution to destroy both surface and hidden bacteria. The wood should then be thoroughly dried, following which the first coat of polyurethane should be applied. This will usually be soaked up completely by the wood, but after a few hours it will form a base for the second coat. This coat will very often be soaked up again, but having allowed it to dry out, if a third liberal coat is applied the wood should end up with a glazed finish which will resist chipping or extremes of heat and which is smooth, impervious and capable of being readily cleaned. In coating table legs, care should be taken to apply the varnish to the surface in contact with the floor, otherwise moisture may be drawn up the wood and in turn may cause the varnish to peel.

There is an exception to the general rule relating to the use of wood. This is where the traditional chopping block is concerned. Although a more desirable synthetic alternative is available, the traditional block is still considered to be an essential piece of equipment by many.

Chopping blocks

These are usually made of a denser, heavier type of wood which is less absorbent than soft wood. To give it additional strength, so that it will not split along the grain, the block is made up of a series of squares of wood which are bonded together. Although it may be dense, the fact that it is wood means that extra special care should be taken with regard to maintenance and cleaning, particularly as it is going to receive heavy treatment from knives and cleavers which, inevitably, are going to create potential harbourages for dirt and bacteria.

The important point about cleaning a block is to ensure, first of all, that as smooth a surface as possible is maintained so that dirt is not trapped unnecessarily. Having cleaned away visible dirt with a scraper and wire brush, it is then necessary to apply a disinfectant solution which will soak into the block and destroy any bacteria which have penetrated into the body of the wood and where they might multiply and provide a reservoir of infection.

Although chopping blocks are usually thick and will withstand

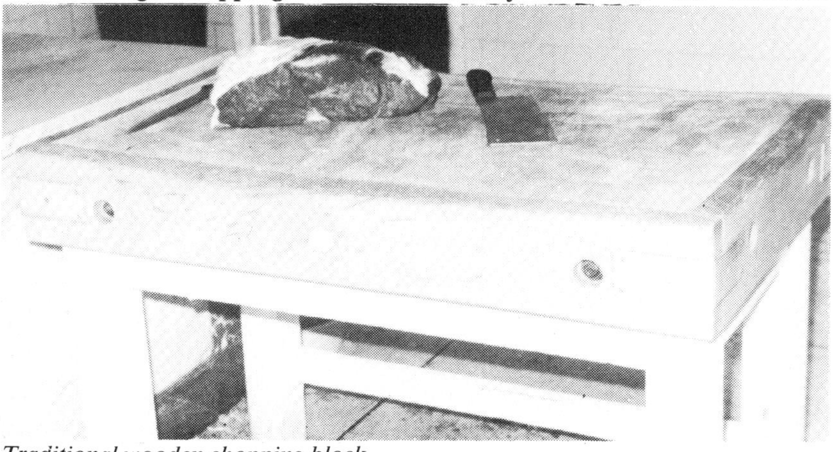

Traditional wooden chopping block

considerable wear, there comes a time when the surface has worn too much to enable proper cleaning. The normal practice is to turn the block over and use the reverse side which is similarly constructed. It may be possible, where there is sufficient thickness, for a specialist firm to remove the top layer of wood to leave a smooth surface.

Cutting boards

Metal preparation tables will last for years if properly used, but one of the problems often encountered in catering premises is that handlers abuse the surface by using it for cutting or chopping to the extent that it becomes scored or broken. In this condition, it is bound to provide a harbourage for bacteria. Neither stainless steel nor laminated nor formica type surfaces are suitable for cutting or chopping. Chopping should always be confined to a chopping block, while cutting should always be carried out on a special cutting board. Although some hardwood cutting boards are available, the more modern composition or rubber based boards are better because they do not crack and most types can be put into boiling water to sterilise them. All boards inevitably become scored at some stage and when this happens the board should be discarded; although in some cases, manufacturers are able to remove the thin upper layer which is most affected to leave a new smooth cutting surface.

Some composition boards do not withstand high water temperatures readily, in which case they should be steeped in a disinfectant solution for cleaning purposes.

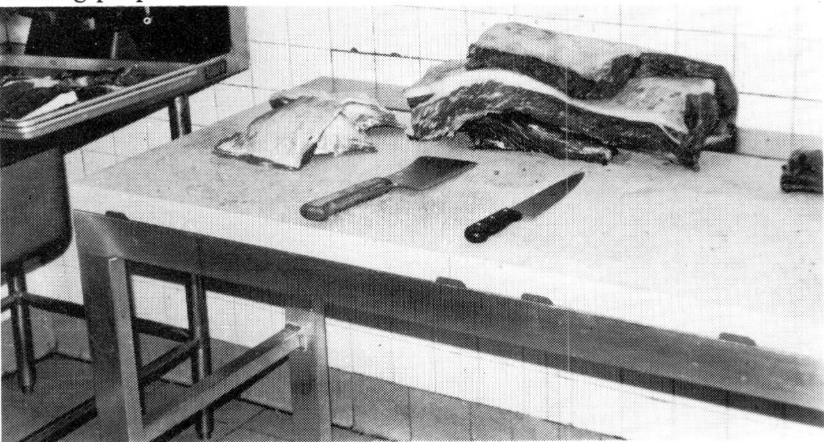

Modern synthetic chopping table (James Whitside & co.)

The food handler must be familiar with the dangers from cross-contamination, that is the transfer of infection from one food onto equipment or hands followed by the further transfer from that equipment or those hands onto a second food. There is a very high incidence of cross-contamination when using cutting boards which have been used for a variety of foods without adequate cleaning in between and very special care should be taken to ensure that boards are well maintained and thoroughly cleaned between use. On no account should the same cutting board and knives be used for both raw and cooked foods.

Food preparation surfaces

The choice of surface on which food is to be prepared is vitally important. Failure to ensure a suitable material may provide a dangerous breeding ground for bacteria.

For the reasons outlined earlier, wood should not be used, although it may be used as a base for another surface. For example, a wooden table may be covered with a non-absorbent material such as stainless steel or plastic laminate, both of which provide an excellent surface. Where this is done, however, care should be taken to ensure that there are no hidden gaps between the surface and the table which might harbour dirt. Edges, particularly, should be formed so that water and food scraps cannot work underneath.

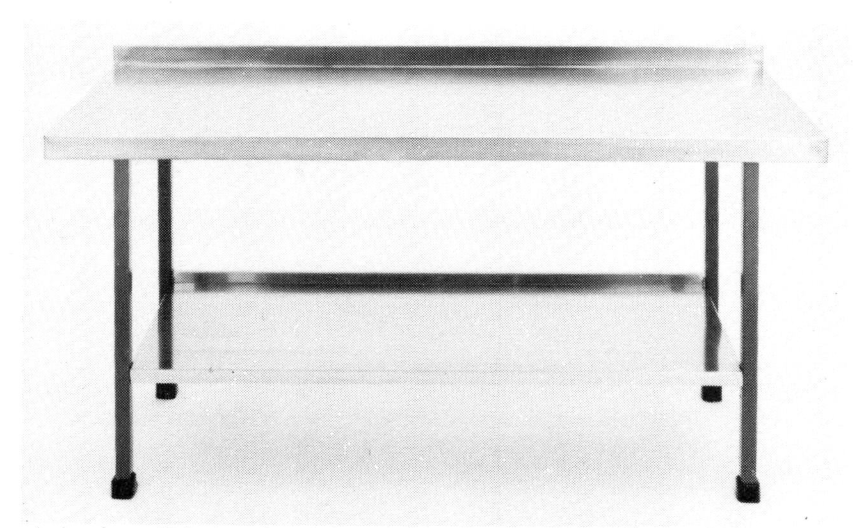

A simple, well-designed, stainless steel preparation table (Sissons of Sheffield)

The design of tables has improved considerably over the past few years with a tendency to simplify as much as possible to permit easy cleaning. Stainless steel tables are the best because they do not rust and with their welded seams, eliminate unwanted cracks or open joints. Sealed tubular legs are preferable to angular iron ones because again they eliminate corners in which dirt collects. Tables with open sides and without drawers are best because likewise they provide less opportunity for dirt to accumulate. If drawers are necessary, they should be of rust-proof metal and easily removable to allow thorough cleaning. Wooden drawers should not be encouraged but where they exist, they may be made acceptable by cleaning and sealing, as described above, with polyurethane varnish.

Slicing machines

Effective cleaning of these is especially important because of the risk of cross-contamination of foods. The design of slicers has improved considerably over the past few years, but by virtue of their winding gear and other moving parts as well as the cutting edge itself, all of which necessitate some type of covering or shield, the design is fairly complicated with numerous potential sites for dirt and bacteria to collect if the machine is neglected.

Good food practices should apply in the use of the machine and, for example, cooked meats should never be placed on a machine where raw meat may have previously been sliced without it being thoroughly cleaned first. Failure to do so may give rise to cross-contamination between the foods.

In choosing the best slicer for the job, having agreed on the size, decided whether it is to be manually or electrically operated, and checked that the necessary safety features have been incorporated to protect the operator, the best model will be that where the blade and blade housing can be readily dismantled for easy cleaning. The blade must be cleaned daily, but it may also need to be cleaned between cutting various foods and a few simple wing nuts are preferable to a complicated system of nuts and bolts for releasing covers. Thorough cleaning of the following parts is essential: the blade, carriageway, and hand-guard as well as the blade casing, which may become contaminated by pieces of food being thrown from the blade when rotating.

Most machines are made of stainless steel or aluminium. These are easily kept clean and have the advantage over metals which are enamelled, by not chipping or requiring periodic painting.

Machines tend to have the minimum number of oil or grease points but care should be taken to ensure that only oil recommended by the manufacturer is used. This will normally be vegetable oil based and certainly non-toxic.

Where electrically-powered slicers are used, they should be situated near a power point to avoid using long leads. Leads in any case should be securely fixed to the wall and not allowed to trail across the floor or equipment.

Cookers

These are inevitably going to become soiled with food particles, which may well become baked onto the sides or beneath burners. Although sufficiently high temperatures may be applied which will kill off most bacteria in the cooking process, some contamination may occur through particles dropping into the food from the accumulation that has been allowed to remain. The debris will also provide a source of food for insects and rodents.

Although a thorough and regular cleaning programme must be applied with cooking ranges, the design can make this routine less arduous. Cookers should be simple in construction with large

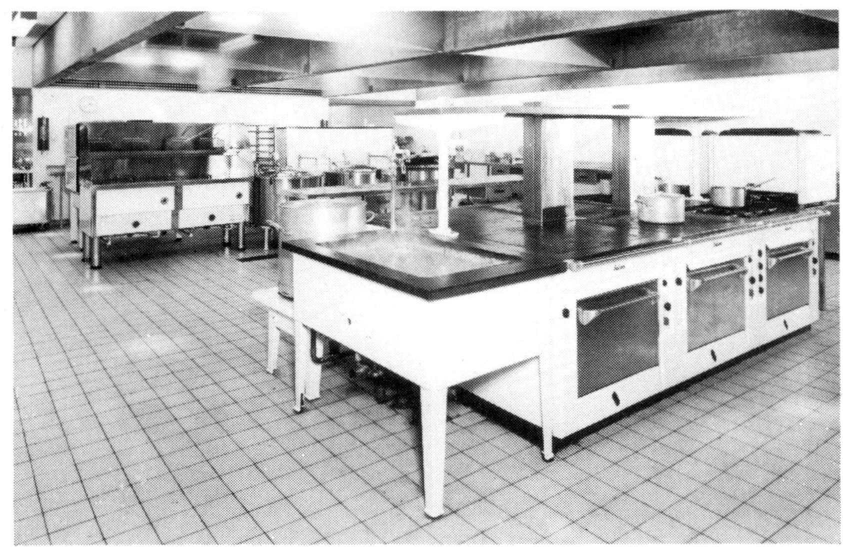

Large "island" cooking range (W. M. Still & Sons Ltd)

uncomplicated surfaces rather than more fanciful designs which will make cleaning difficult. Preference should be given to stainless steel construction over enamelled metal.

The inside surfaces should be easily removable and spillage plates below heating rings should also be readily accessible for cleaning purposes.

Cooking ranges should be raised 10-15 cm (4-6 in) off the ground to allow easy cleaning. If they are near the walls, they should be situated a sufficient distance away to enable a person to reach behind when cleaning. Cookers that are situated on an island site, have the advantage of being able to be cleaned "all-round".

The storage of fuel in most cases does not present a problem, but in the case of solid fuel cooking ranges, care should be taken to ensure that the minimum dust is created when loading the hopper. Fuel must never be stored in the food area.

Gas ranges should be serviced periodically to check on the efficiency of the burners which sometimes become partially blocked by food particles. In the case of oil and solid fuel ranges, checks should be made of flues to ensure that they are clean and free from obstruction.

Heating cabinets and ovens

These are of metal construction. In recent years, there have been moves to make cleaning that much easier through eliminating hidden areas and difficult corners. The best ovens are those which permit one to reach every part with ease. Doors are either hinged or sliding. While the latter are more convenient in that one does not need an "opening" area for the door, problems can arise through dust collecting in the tracks.

Cabinets and ovens should be raised 10-15 cm (4-6 in) off the ground to permit easy cleaning. Regular cleaning of the equipment itself is necessary to prevent any spillage becoming caked, which will be that much more difficult to remove later.

Mincing machines

The majority of catering establishments, as well as butchers and some grocers, will use a mincer for reducing the size of meat or vegetables. Most mincers are of metal and consist of a worm drive which pushes the food on to and through a series of perforated discs which determine the final size of the food. The machines are either manually or electrically driven and demand special attention because of the danger of food particles becoming lodged in the worm and associated mechanism.

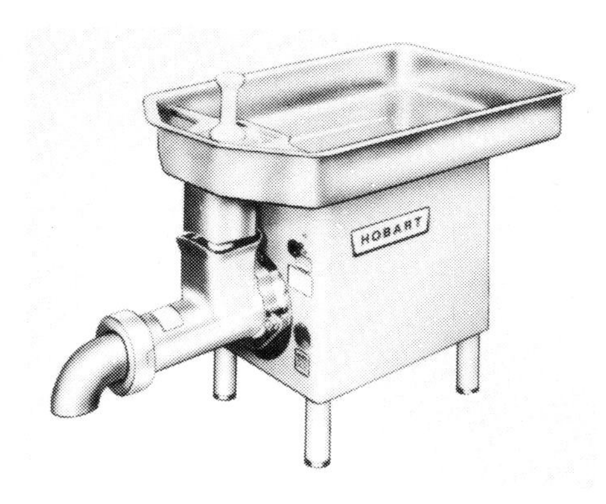

Modern mincing machine (Hobart Manufacturing Co. Ltd)

Modern mincers are designed to facilitate easy cleaning by allowing the easy removal of the worm and mincing discs through one or two simple wing nuts. The actual reception hopper should be so shaped to eliminate unnecessary corners in which food may lodge. Once dismantled, all those parts that come into contact with the food should be thoroughly cleaned and steeped in a disinfectant solution.

An important point here, this applies to all hand operated machinery, care should be taken to ensure that all handles are equally well cleaned. Plastic handles or grips are preferable to wood and the handles should be steeped in a disinfectant solution to ensure that the hidden area beneath the handle is adequately cleaned.

Potato peelers

These require special attention because inevitably they will collect dirt from the potatoes, either on the scraper discs or in the main wash tanks. They should be thoroughly cleaned at the end of each working day to ensure that peelings and dirt do not accumulate, decompose and attract pests.

Chippers

These are often neglected because of the inherent difficulty in cleaning the actual slicing grids. The grids and associated mechanism, which should be of stainless steel, must be dismantled and thoroughly cleaned at the end of each working day to ensure that there is no accumulation of food particles.

Beer and other drink dispensing machines

Most of the traditional hand-pulls in public houses have been replaced by pressurised systems, whereby independent gas cylingers force the liquid from the kegs or tanks through pipes to the taps at the bar or counter. Special controls ensure that the gas used is safe and breweries take great care to ensure that the barrels themselves are clean.This has been made much easier since the introduction of metal barrels to replace those made of wood.

Although stainless metal pipework is still used, transparent plastic piping is being installed to an increasing extent both because of its lower cost and because it can be examined more readily for signs of dirt. Pipework should be regularly cleaned by flushing through with an approved disinfecting agent, followed by a rinse with clean, hot water.

Mixing machines

Mixers may be used for a variety of different foods and thorough cleaning, especially of the bowl and paddles, is necessary between different foods. Most commercial models are relatively heavy and because of the almost inevitable problems with spillage during mixing or from flour dust, they should be fitted with rollers to allow easy removal for cleaning. If placed on tables they should be slightly raised to permit effective cleaning underneath. Electricity supply cables should be dealt with as for slicing machines. Care is essential to ensure that articles of clothing do not become entangled with the paddles during operation.

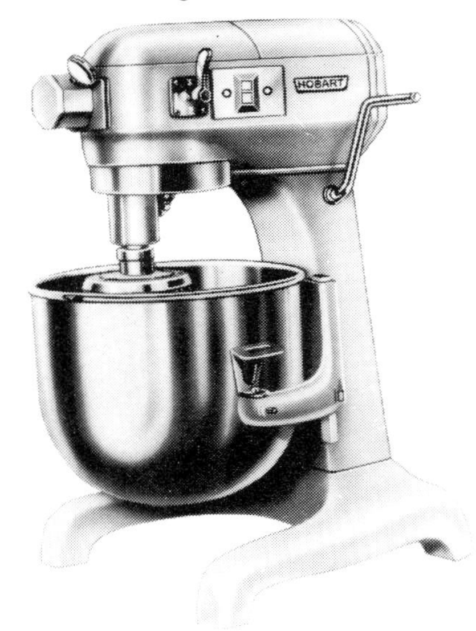

Commercial food mixer (Hobart Manufacturing Co. Ltd)

Although early models used wooden paddles, these have been replaced with various designs made from stainless steel or aluminium which have the advantage of being stronger and much easier to keep clean. Bowls and containers, depending on their size, are available in pyrex or stainless steel and provided they are kept in good condition, present few problems.

Ice-cream (Soft) machines

These also require special attention, not only because of the nature of the food, but also because of the intricate pipe-work and valves employed, which can provide a harbourage for bacteria if not properly cleaned. Although pipework and the main tank are usually of stainless steel, they must be kept clean and all pipes, taps and valves should be taken apart at the end of each day, washed and steeped in disinfectant solution, then rinsed with clean water.

Ice-cream should not remain in the machine overnight. Care should be taken not to remove drips from the tap with, for example, a wiping cloth which may itself contaminate the tap and ice-cream.

Sinks

The Food Hygiene Regulations, 1970, require that, in all food premises where open food is handled, sinks or other washing facilities must be provided for washing food and equipment. These must be provided with hot and cold water supplies or hot water at a suitably controlled temperature. In planning washing facilities, care should be taken to ensure that the hot water tank is capable of maintaining sufficient supplies at a suitable temperature.

Regard should be had to maximum loads when fixing the capacity of the tank and the size of heater to be used. Both will have a marked bearing on how efficiently staff work because with only tepid water they will take twice as long to do a cleaning job than with hot water, besides which only hot water will effectively remove grease deposits. (See Chapter 5.)

Sinks should ideally be manufactured in high quality stainless steel (18/8) as this metal is stain resistant, rust resistant, and capable of withstanding considerable misuse. Galvanised sinks, enamel sinks and glazed stoneware sinks are all inferior, the latter two being particularly prone to chipping and consequently failing to provide a smooth, impervious surface. Whilst stainless steel is more expensive to install initially, it is a far better investment in the long term. A brief word about plumbing services might be appropriate at this juncture.

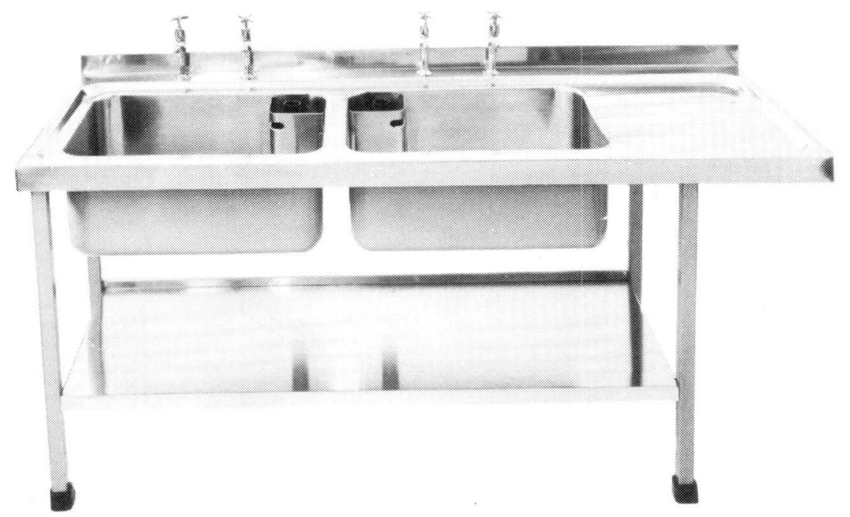

Stainless steel double sink unit (Sissons of Sheffield)

Modern plumbing materials include unplasticised polyvinylchloride (UPVC), copper and cast iron, with a tendency to use the former in place of the more traditional materials. This is partly because of initial cost and partly because of the less skilled plumbing work necessary with UPVC. It should, however, be noted that copper and cast iron withstand high temperatures and accidental damage far more successfully and should be used in preference to UPVC in food premises.

Hand washing facilities

Washhand basins should be of stainless steel or glazed vitreous ware and should be supplied with hot and cold water, a plastic nailbrush, soap or other detergent, and suitable means for hand drying. Although the Food Hygiene Regulations, 1970, refer to washhand basins, in practice the caterer will be wise to ensure that he installs a basin which is slightly larger in size to enable handlers to wash their wrists and forearms which may become soiled as well. The use of a larger basin also helps to prevent splashing onto the floor. This subject is covered in greater detail in Chapter 8.

Utensils

It is easy for any utensil to become a vehicle for the transfer of infection. Knives, choppers, boning tools, whisks and spoons all have access to a wide variety of foods as well as to man himself and, for this reason, special care is important. The condition of utensils must be maintained not only to ensure that they are safe — bearing in mind that a blunt knife is potentially far more dangerous than a sharp one — but also to enable it to be thoroughly cleaned. Whilst the working parts of most equipment are of metal and present few problems, some by virtue of their design do create difficulties. For example, whisks may be of metal but because of their intricate design may make cleaning difficult. Hence it is much better to choose a model which can be effectively cleaned rather than one which has hidden areas where food might lodge.

Wooden handles for utensils are slowly being replaced by plastic ones which are non-absorbent and are easily moulded about the metal part to eliminate hidden spaces for dirt and bacteria to accumulate. Although there was early opposition to plastic handles by the industry on the grounds of their being difficult to grip, modern design has produced handles which are both non-slip and easy to clean.

Wooden spoons should be discouraged because they are absorbent and quickly become worn and cracked. They are difficult to clean effectively and should be replaced with plastic or metal, the former being equally acceptable for use in connection with non-stick appliances.

Although referred to in the chapter dealing with the storage of food, the need for trays and containers to be of suitable material is important. As a general rule, wood should not be used because of the difficulty in

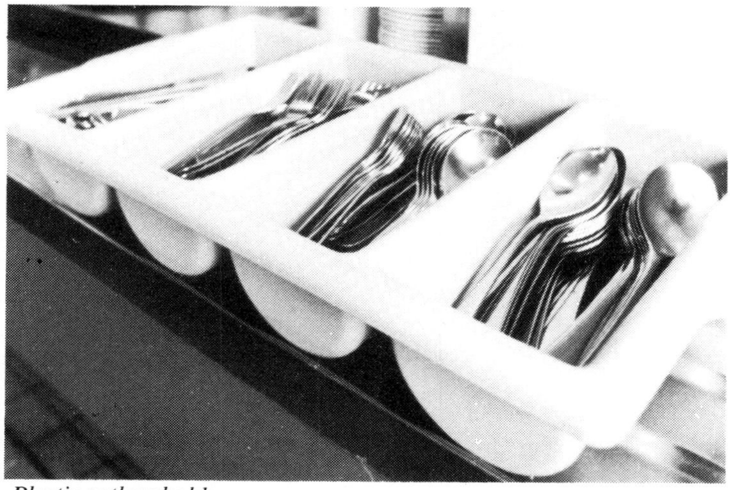

Plastic cutlery holder

cleaning it efficiently. Plastic, polythene and metal are preferable because they are non-absorbent, can be easily cleaned and can be so designed and constructed to eliminate hidden harbourage for dirt.

Containers used for the storage of utensils such as knives, forks and spoons should be of plastic or metal construction and should be so designed as to eliminate corners in which dirt might accumulate. Nests of individual pockets are available in plastic or metal and are designed so that each pocket is "U" shaped. These make cleaning easier and enable utensils to be handled more quickly and safely.

Tin openers require special care, particularly table-mounted models. These can become very dirty as a result of the grease used to lubricate the column forming an accumulation with food particles. The piercing edge itself can become contaminated and, unless cleaned between use, could give rise to contamination between foods. The most effective method of cleaning is to remove the entire opener and immerse it in hot deteregent and water which will remove all the grease and debris. The track, which is usually set on the table, can then be either steam-cleaned or brushed with a hot soda solution.

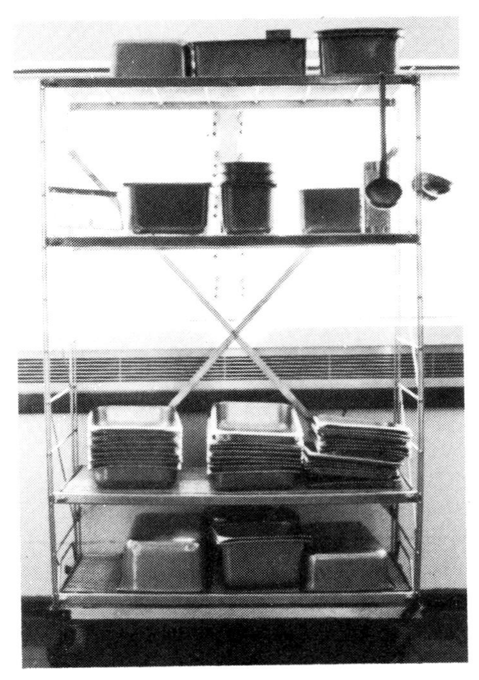

Mobile pan and utensil rack

The common habit of keeping knives on open racks screwed to the kitchen wall should not be encouraged because they are difficult to keep clean and can also be dangerous.

Saucepans, pots and other similar cooking containers will invariably be of metal. Accumulations of dirt, including that on the outside, should be removed and each appliance should be regularly checked to ensure that there are no cracks which might harbour dirt. Handles should also be regularly checked to ensure that they are secure for carrying and lifting.

Storage

The storage of equipment needs careful consideration. Pots and pans may be stacked upside-down on metal racks near the cooking area. The racks should be mounted on castors to allow them to be moved. The racks themselves, of course, should be regularly cleaned.

Plates and dishes are best stored on either metal or formica-covered shelves in cupboards. They should not be placed on cloths or sponge sheeting which, although intended to provide a less damaging surface, can become a source of contamination.

All those utensils which contain or are plated with metal containing lead or any other potentially harmful metal or chemical should not be used. Any coated utensil where the covering has broken or worn, should be either discarded or replated.

Chipped or damaged plates, cups or other crockery should be discarded, because of the danger from bacteria which may be present in the cracks.

Chapter 5

CLEANSING TECHNIQUES

By now the reader will have gathered, if he or she didn't already know, that food hygiene is all about cleanliness, and it is appropriate to examine the way in which a state of cleanliness can be achieved. As with most problems, there are a number of different aspects which need to be considered in order to obtain the best results: the nature of the equipment, its construction and situation, the type of dirt to be removed, the time available, the cleaning materials, cleaning equipment and the staff available to complete the task, are all important considerations. Each of these points will be considered, but first let us examine the various types of cleaning materials available and their advantages and disadvantages.

Soap
Manufactured from animal and vegetable oil in either hard tablet form or liquid gel. It frequently forms a scum when used in hard water supplies and is not very efficient at removing bacteria. It is mainly used for personal hygiene.

Washing cream
Made from pure vegetable oils, the cream is rubbed well into the hands prior to wetting and is very efficient, even in hard water areas, at a much lower cost than hard or liquid soaps.

Synthetic detergents
Detergents are chemicals which are capable of dissolving grease, oil and dirt into suspension in water.

1. Anionic (negative charged) detergents comprise the bulk of the common liquid and powder household detergents, used for clothes' washing and dishwashing.
2. Nonionic (neutral) detergents are particularly useful in hard water areas, as they have less tendency to foam and dissolve mineral oils extremely efficiently.
3. Cationic (positive charged) detergents are complex chemicals which are capable of dissolving grease. They also provide a sterilising effect on the surface of the material being cleansed.

Disinfectants
These are chemicals which have germ-destroying properties of a proven standard (B.S. 2462:1961). They may also be called sanitizers, germicides, bactericides or sterilants. They may be used in conjunction with detergents, but beware of cheap, "pine" smelling solutions which are seldom of the required quality. Care must be taken to avoid mixing anionic disinfectants with cationic detergents.

Hypochlorites (bleach) and quaternary ammonium compounds are two examples of disinfectants which are currently available for use as sanitizers but which require special precautions to prevent misuse.

One problem does confront the purchaser of detergents and disinfectants, and that relates to the wide choice and price differentials. The Government has not, so far, produced a list of approved chemicals for the catering industry, despite the presence of a list for the dairy industry. In consequence there are a number of cheap chemicals on the market that are, frankly, little more than coloured liquid and completely useless. It is a false economy to purchase such products — always look for the well-known household names as their substantial reputations have been proven. A further check can be made to see whether the relevant British Standard Specification number is quoted on the label.

Scouring powders
These cleaning materials combine a detergent with an abrasive and frequently a hypochlorite to assist with the removal of hardened food deposits in cooking utensils. Care should be taken to avoid damaging surfaces by over-zealous cleaning with coarse powders. The use of oven cleaners should be unnecessary if routine cleaning of ovens is carried out. A weak solution of bicarbonate of soda should be used to coat the inside surfaces, as this dries on and absorbs the fat from the food subsequently cooked in the oven.

Floor cleaners and polishes

A variety of liquid and wax-based cleansers and polishes are marketed to remove dirt and provide a shiny, even a non-slip, surface to tiles, stone, vinyl and synthetic flooring found in food premises.

With the wide range of chemicals available for use, it is important to obtain the correct product for the job, to follow the instructions carefully and to check with the supplier or manufacturer if in doubt. Never mix dissimilar chemicals and only use at the correct dilution rates. Weak solutions are not effective, while strong solutions are not necessarily more effective and are merely wasteful of chemical.

Cleaning equipment

As with chemicals, there is a variety of equipment available for use in catering premises, ranging from disposable cloths to dish-washing machines, and some of this equipment will be specifically discussed later.

Dealing with the cleansing of surfaces first, everyone is familiar with the

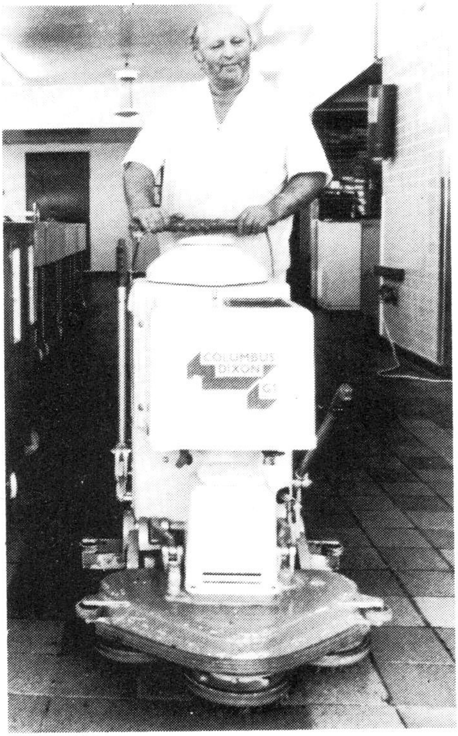

A mechanical floor cleaner

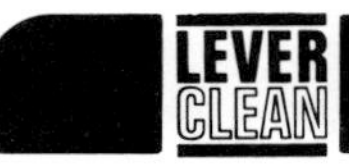

CLEANLINESS RECORD *from*
Lever Industrial Limited

COMPANY ....

ADDRESS (or Branch) ....

SHEET No.

DATE

Copyright

✓ SATISFACTORY / ✗ REQUIRES ATTENTION	Date of Inspection					
FOOD STORAGE						
Walls/Windows						
Floor						
Shelves/Racks						
Containers/Bins						
PREPARATION						
Walls/Windows						
Floor						
Mixers						
Slicers						
Cooking utensils						
Cookers						
Working surfaces						
Meat blocks						
Refrigerator						
Cupboards/Racks						
Swabbing cloths						
Fish range						
Canopies						
Sinks/Drainage						
SERVERY						
Cups/Saucers						
Plates						
Cutlery						
Glassware						
Servers						
Trays						
Plate separators						
Hotplates						
Cupboards/Racks						
Tea urns						
Tea/Coffee pots						

✓ SATISFACTORY / ✗ REQUIRES ATTENTION	Date of Inspection					
SERVERY—cont.						
Swabbing cloths						
Food Display cabinets						
Trolleys						
Condiment containers						
WASHING UP						
Sinks—Washing						
Sinks—Sterilizing						
Draining boards						
Dishcloths						
Drying cloths						
MACHINE						
Interior						
Exterior						
Wash jets/Brushes						
Rinse jets						
Curtains						
Overflows						
Trays/Racks						
Drainage						
STAFF						
Overalls etc.						
Hands						
DINING (1)						
Tables/Chairs						
Linen						
Floor/Carpets						
Walls/Windows						

✓ SATISFACTORY / ✗ REQUIRES ATTENTION	Date of Inspection					
DINING (2)						
Tables/Chairs						
Linen						
Floor/Carpets						
Walls/Windows						
DINING (3) **(or Licensed)**						
Tables/Chairs						
Linen						
Floor/Carpets						
Walls/Windows						
Bar counter						
Glass sinks/Machine						
Cellar floor/Sump						
TOILETS (Public)						
Wash basins						
Towels						
Toilets/Urinals						
Floor/Walls/Fittings						
TOILETS (Staff)						
Wash basins						
Towels						
Toilets/Urinals						
Floor/Walls/Fittings						
GENERAL						
Drains						
Wastepipes						
Waste bins						

The "Lever Clean" record chart (Lever Industrial Ltd)

mop and bucket. These are not recommended but, if they have to be used, the mop requires daily washing and drying or soaking in a disinfectant solution. The bucket can be the breeding-ground for various bacteria unless kept clean and dry. Sponge mops are more effective and hygienic for floor cleaning but must be cleaned daily.

Mechanical scrubbing machines are efficient if used as instructed, but again special attention should be paid to cleaning and storing the brushes and the machinery or they will act as reservoirs for bacteria. It is essential to dry the equipment before storage, even over-night storage.

The use of dish cloths and floor cloths should be discouraged. Rather disposable paper or non-woven fabrics should be used which can be used for one cleaning job and then discarded. In this way the risk of spreading dirt and bacteria is minimised.

Planning cleansing

Before examining the particular cleansing techniques employed in catering, it is necessary to emphasise the importance of regular cleaning. It is rarely carried out enthusiastically and, by tradition, is a job done by the trainees or the lowest grade of staff. The importance of cleaning has always been underestimated and, not unnaturally, the authors place a great deal of importance on the thorough cleaning of premises and equipment. To "lead by example" is a good principle for the proprietor or manager, because staff respond to the "boss" who is prepared to undertake the menial tasks in order to keep the equipment wholesome. There can be no excuse for the accumulations of grease and dirt frequently seen in some catering premises, if one follows the clean-up-as-you-go rule. This is particularly true of preparation surfaces and cooking equipment.

The premises, i.e., floors, walls, ceilings and equipment, will have to receive regular cleaning and this is where a planned routine will be invaluable. The building or department should be divided up into rooms or areas and a separate schedule prepared for each part. Every detail of the premises, including windows, outside gullies, drains, ventilation system, sanitary accommodation and offices, should be listed. The frequency of cleaning and the method and materials should be specified. Staff should be involved in the discussions on their particular cleaning responsibilities to stimulate interest and the management should carry out regular inspections to ensure a satisfactory standard is maintained. Special training in the techniques should be undertaken and, in larger establishments, records of inspections should be kept. Cleaning should be recognised as a scientific management technique.

Specialist cleaning contractors are now available to undertake heavy duty cleaning of catering premises on a routine basis. Steam or chemical solutions are used to remove encrusted material but, once the original surface has been restored, it is usually possible to maintain it by daily cleansing. Exceptions to this are the cleaning of ventilation ducting fans, degreasing of specialist equipment, servicing of grease gullies, drains and similar equipment. Staff usually respond to the incentive of working in clean premises, but the highest standards can only be achieved by constant effort on a systematic programme.

In order to provide for efficient, labour-saving cleaning routines, it is necessary to examine the design of premises and equipment and to introduce specifications which incorporate all the advantages and none of the disadvantages which modern materials can produce. Some design details will be examined in the following notes which highlight various parts of a cleaning operation.

Hot water supply

Without question the first fundamental in any cleaning operation is the availability of plentiful supplies of hot water. This is not always found in catering premises, but it is absolutely essential and a legal requirement. Hot water systems are available from a variety of sources and heaters, the most efficient being via a central boiler, the poorest from a small sink-type element heater which does not provide constant hot water.

Floors

Special attention must be given to floors because of the obvious dangers which wet, slippery or greasy surfaces present to staff. Spillages must be removed immediately and the use of sawdust or cardboard should be prohibited as both encourage dirty conditions despite the alleged safety claims. Daily cleaning of floors, particularly floor channels, grids, gulleys and wall/floor junctions, behind ovens, underneath tables and cupboards is essential. The use of coving at the wall/floor junction assists in cleaning, as does the use of round legs on equipment, moveable equipment or cantilevered fittings.

Walls

These should be finished with glazed tiles, polypropelene welded sheeting or a similar smooth impervious material which incorporates the advantages of a non-absorbent, easily-cleaned surface with lower maintenance costs. Routine cleaning with hot detergent water is sufficient without the additional decorating costs which would be incurred with plastered walls.

Lighting

Windows should, of course, be subject to regular cleaning both inside and out in order to obtain maximum benefit from natural lighting. Many catering premises have to rely on artificial lighting to a large extent and it should be emphasised that this produces inferior working conditions. Light fittings need to be kept clean, especially the diffusers on fluorescent tubes. If the fittings are suspended, routine cleaning of the upper surfaces should be undertaken as these attract dirt and dust.

Freezers and refrigerators

These vital pieces of modern catering equipment are frequently abused. It is essential to defrost them regularly and at the same time to clean them thoroughly using detergent and hot water. Walk-in freezers or cold rooms should be washed out weekly to avoid accumulations of dirt and debris on the floor.

Ventilation

An essential component in almost all kitchens, whether in the form of a simple extract fan or a fully ducted air conditioning system. The design of many ventilation systems is inferior, leaving too many dust and dirt collecting surfaces which require regular cleansing. Filters and ductwork need inspecting every fourteen days because of the fire risk inherent in grease and dirt. Anti-drip channels need special attention as do the special ventilation systems provided to deep-frying pans or ranges.

Preparation equipment

The food preparation stage is where the highest standards of hygiene need to be observed and therefore equipment and working surfaces need to be spotlessly clean. This means that equipment must be kept in good condition and cleaned after every use to avoid cross contamination. Suitable detergent/disinfectant solutions, not phenolic disinfectants which will taint food, should be employed and the surface thoroughly dried with a clean disposable cloth after use. This is especially important between use for preparing raw food and cooked food, particularly meat, fish or dairy products. Wiping the surfaces with a re-usable cloth is not acceptable as this merely transfers the contamination.

Special attention should be given to the regular cleaning of food slicers and mincers (remember the Aberdeen typhoid outbreak in 1966), not overlooking the prohibition on untrained employees under eighteen years of age. Such equipment should be carefully dismantled to ensure thorough cleaning of all parts.

Sinks and washing-up

Ideally all crockery and cutlery should be machine-washed, and this principle is discussed in detail later on. It is appreciated that many premises will continue to hand-wash not only crocks but also pots and pans, so a detailed examination of the correct procedures is necessary.

The sinks themselves should be of stainless steel construction incorporating draining boards and, ideally, a sink waste grinder. The use of enamel or glazed stoneware sinks is inadvisable because of their vulnerability to chipping or cracking which leaves an unhygienic surface. The sinks and fittings must be thoroughly cleaned after use with a fresh disinfectant solution.

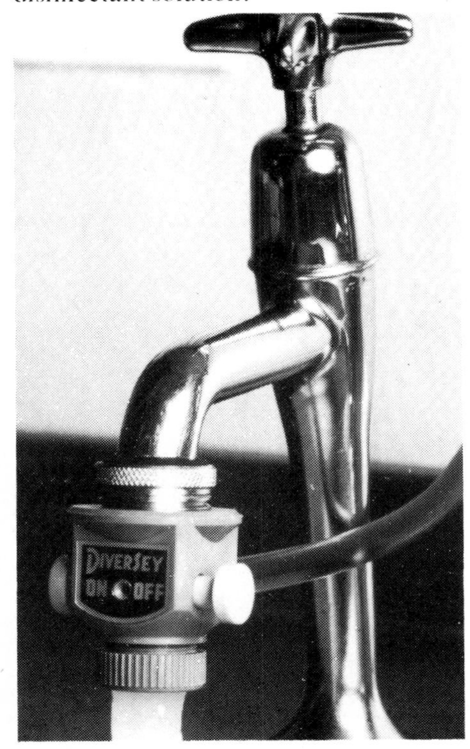

Detergent tap proportioner (Diversey Ltd)

One sink should be used to wash the crockery and cutlery in a suitable detergent solution in order to remove dirt and grease or fat. This solution may be controlled by the use of a tap proportioner connected to a drum of detergent, so that a measured supply of detergent automatically mixes with the water in the sink. Clean nylon brushes should be used but not dishcloths. The water should be regularly changed and maintained at 60°C (140°F).

The equipment should then be transferred for at least one minute to the rinsing sink, containing clean water at 82°C (180°F), which has the effect of destroying any remaining bacteria. As the hands will not withstand such temperatures, rubber gloves or baskets will be necessary.

Once cleaned and rinsed, the crockery, cutlery, etc. should be either air-dried, heat-dried or hand-dried using disposable paper towelling. Tea towels should not be used, even if freshly laundered each day, because of the risk of cross contamination which would defeat the object of disinfection.

Plates should be thoroughly dried before stacking. Pots and utensils should be dried before storage. All equipment should then be stored in closed cupboards to reduce the risk of contamination from dust and dirt. Chipped, cracked, stained or broken items should be discarded immediately.

Washing by machine

Dish-washing machines are expensive pieces of equipment, especially if one accepts the manufacturers' advice to use softened water for best results. There is little doubt that the industrial models provide an efficient labour-saving service to cope with that chore which is one of the least popular in the kitchen. Most machines give a wash and rinse cycle similar to the technique described above, but their biggest fault is their inability to remove dried or encrusted dirt and grease effectively. Some pre-washing is usually necessary when stacking the crockery and cutlery in the trays. Another point to note is that manual washing-up facilities will still have to be available in the event of a machine breakdown.

The use of glass-washing equipment is becoming increasingly popular in public houses and bars of all types. Several models are available with variations on the principle of revolving rubber spikes and jets of hot water. These machines are vastly superior to the old method of a quick rinse under the bar counter in tepid dirty water and a quick rub round with a damp tea cloth! A glass-cleaning cloth is still sometimes found necessary to "polish" the glass and remove the obstinate lipstick, but the bacteria on the average glass has to be "seen" to be believed. There is a lot to be said

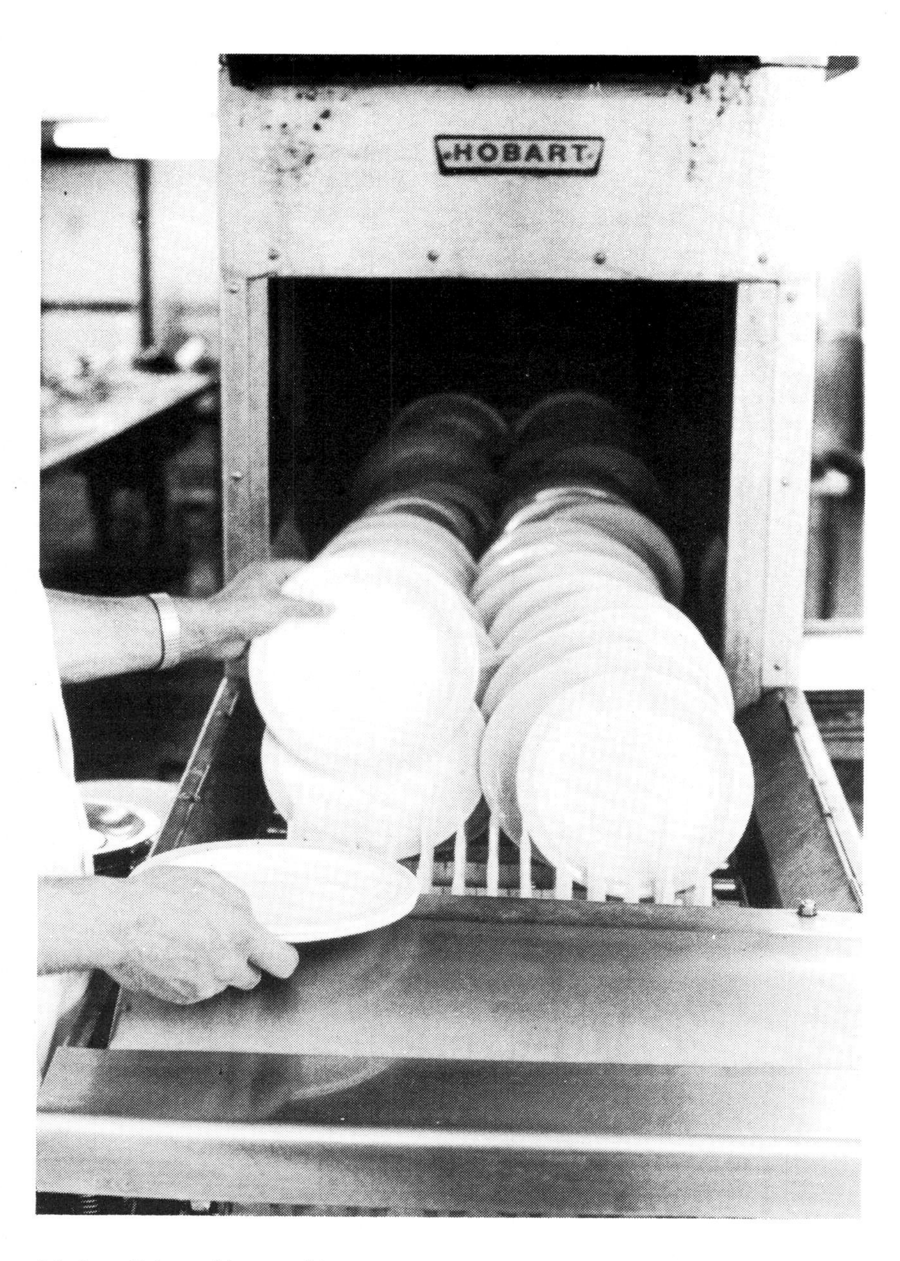

Modern dish-washing machine

for the Scottish regulations which forbid a publican to serve a fresh drink in a used glass (even one's own!). Freshly-laundered glass cloths, or preferably paper cloths, should be used, and a suitable detergent/ disinfectant added to the hot water.

A final comment on the cleaning of silverware, still to be found in use in the more salubrious establishments, take care not to recontaminate the cutlery with dirty hands!

Sanitary accommodation

Thorough cleaning is necessary using proper disinfectant solutions. This extends not only to the compartments and the closet and basins, but also to the associated equipment such as chains, levers, door handles and light switches.

Refuse storage

Although not technically a subject requiring to be discussed in this chapter, refuse storage nevertheless needs to be mentioned because of the cleaning aspects associated with the problem. As previously mentioned, the use of a sink waste-disposal unit is to be preferred or, failing that, a paper or plastic sack system incorporating a sealing device so that the sack can be removed to the refuse storage area both quickly and hygienically. The use of plastic pedal bins and swill bins is to be discouraged because of the hygiene considerations; attraction to insect pests, vermin and smell in particular.

It is advisable to consult the local authority on the preferred methods, because some Councils prohibit the use of sink grinders due to their silting effect on the sewerage system. There is also the question of payment and frequency of the trade refuse collection service which may have a bearing on the final choice of system. All refuse storage areas must be kept neat, clean and tidy by daily attention.

Drainage

Although not a task with which the food handler or kitchen hand will usually be directly involved, it is essential to realise the importance of maintaining clean drainage facilities and to be aware of the potential abuse and expense of dealing with neglected drains. A fundamental rule is that the sink waste gullies should be checked weekly in order to ensure that there is no accumulation of tea leaves or debris likely to create a blockage and overflow. Some gullies may be fitted with special removable baskets to catch such debris from causing more serious trouble, and these baskets may have to be checked daily. Similarly, many catering premises have had grease traps fitted to prevent fat and grease congealing and blocking the drains, and these traps need to be regularly cleaned or the object of providing them is defeated! A strong (5%) bleach solution should be used to clean the waste traps and pipes, twice a week if possible. Manhole covers should be lifted and greased every three months to ensure ease of lifting. These jobs can be undertaken by a servicing contractor who specialises in hygiene services of this nature.

The "Clean" image

This entire book is devoted to various aspects of hygiene and we constantly return to the theme that "Cleanliness sells food". This policy applies to all facets of the catering business, both in front of the customer and behind the scenes. It is important to attend to details such as clean public rooms, clean furniture, napkins and table-cloths, clean cutlery, crockery and condiments — not forgetting the sauce bottles — clean glasses and optics or measures and, above all, clean personnel!

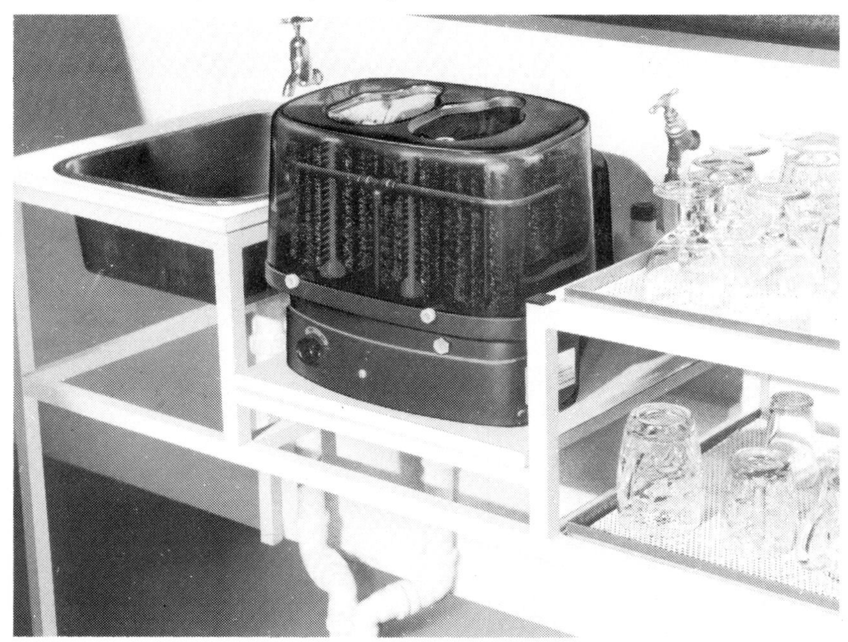

Modern glass-washing machine (Skivvy (U.K.) Ltd)

Chapter 6

THE STORAGE OF FOOD

It has been said that the three golden rules for storing food are to keep it clean, keep it cool and keep it covered. Certainly the way in which food is stored, in any catering premises, can have a marked effect on its quality. Every care should be taken to ensure that the various types of food are stored correctly before, during and after preparation.

It is essential to maintain a proper check on the food by knowing how much of each particular item is present at any one time. Besides being good business management, it means that food is less likely to deteriorate through prolonged storage.

Although it is better from a food hygiene standpoint to maintain limited stocks, so that store rooms do not become congested, modern trading methods often demand that commodities be purchased in bulk. Therefore care should be taken to ensure that food storage and use is properly monitored.

Rotation of stock

Stock rotation — i.e., the control which ensures that older stock is used first — can only be achieved by a check system whereby, as food is received, it is coded. Many manufacturers now mark their products with either an open code which indicates the "sell by" or "death" date to both the retailer and the customer, or a secret code which can be deciphered by the retailer if provided with the key. Retailers sometimes use a colour code to indicate the day/week of delivery, and there are many more complex coding systems. In a catering premises, it is much simpler to use a date system.

The rotation of stock is particularly important with short life or perishable foods which, under normal atmospheric conditions of temperature and humidity, will deteriorate more readily than those foods which have been preserved, whether by canning, drying or freezing. It should be remembered, however, that no food has an unlimited life and even preserved foods require a degree of rotation.

In general terms the siting of store rooms should be such that they are reasonably accessible to delivery men from the outside, while at the same time they should not be too far from the main preparation or sales area. Ideally they should not be exposed to the direct rays of the sun, which could give rise to unacceptably high temperatures.

In large shops and catering premises, particular members of staff should be designated to supervise the stores and, as far as possible, access should be confined to specific persons rather than just anyone. It should be the supervisor's job not only to look after the cleaning of the store and the control of stock, but he should also be responsible for periodically checking the food for signs of insect or other infestation.

Dry food stores

As the name implies, these should be dry and should also be well ventilated and lit. It is not possible to suggest recommended sizes or capacities because much will depend on the type and size of the catering business. Suffice it to say that the larger the area the better. Crowded stores hamper cleaning, can encourage pests and can also make the job of stock control much more difficult.

The same criteria that are applied to other food rooms should apply to the construction, namely that all parts should be capable of being readily cleaned. Walls and floors should be smooth and impervious and, where possible, walls should be coved to the floor for easy cleaning. Ceilings should also be capable of being easily cleaned and in the case of outside stores with corrugated roofs, these should be under drawn with plasterboard or insulation board to prevent condensation.

Effective measures against rodents and insect pests should be taken and all holes and other openings which may allow access should be effectively sealed. This is particularly important around doors and windows and where cables or pipes enter the store.

Although there may be windows, these should always be covered with perforated metal screens which must be properly maintained. Air bricks should be similarly covered with perforated metal or nylon gauze.

If a dry store is to be effective it should be maintained at a cool

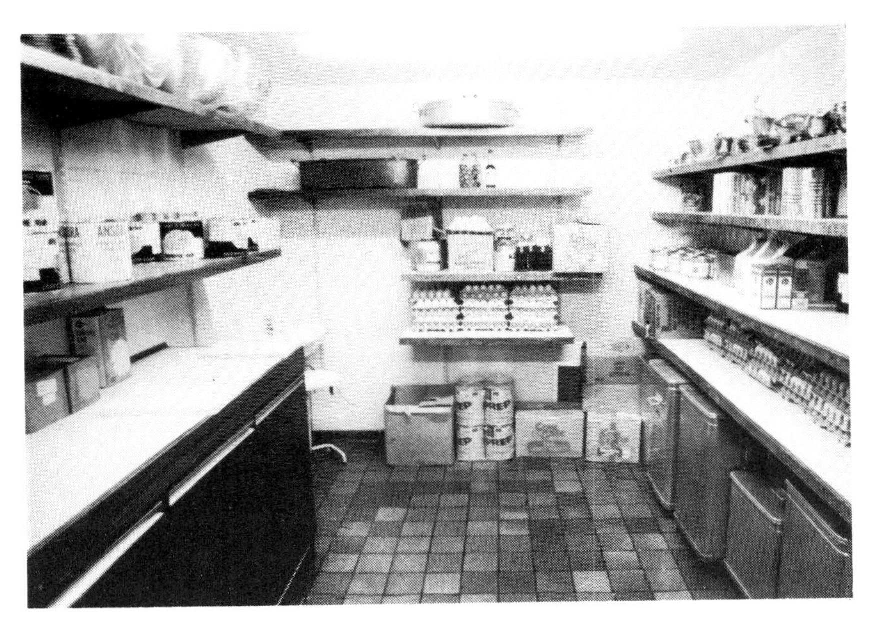

A well-ordered dry store

temperature, around 8°C (44°F). This may be achieved by natural ventilation; although in summer or in an enclosed room, it is best achieved by using a mechanical fan either to exhaust the air into the open or merely to create a movement of air within the room.

Shelving

The fitting out of the store room should be as simple as possible. Most goods will be stored on shelves which can be either open slats or plain wood. In either case they should be smooth and impervious to enable easy cleaning. Wood should be well sanded to give a smooth finish before being gloss painted or varnished to seal it effectively. Metal shelving is being used to an increasing extent. It is of long-term advantage to use rust-proof metals which require far less maintenance.

In fitting shelves, care should be taken to avoid creating corners and voids which will collect dust and dirt and be difficult to clean. Shelves should be removable and should not be so deep as to make the goods towards the back difficult to reach.

Cupboards within the store room should be avoided, but if for any reason they are required, the backs should first be removed so that the units fit closely to the wall. All cupboards and similar units should be capable of being dismantled for cleaning purposes.

The distance between shelves will depend to a large extent on the nature of the goods to be stored, but the lowest shelf should be not less than 75cm (30in) above floor level to permit the storage of bins below. Care should be taken to avoid storage of heavy goods above shoulder height as this creates a safety hazard.

Storage containers

The containers used in a dry store will depend largely on the type of food. Tinned goods can be stored directly on the shelves or, for convenience, in the boxes they are delivered in. However an advantage of removing cans from boxes is that they can be examined for leakage or other defects which may affect other stock.

Some foodstuffs, such as sugar and flour, are often delivered in large quantities and often in paper or polythene bags which are neither strong nor much of a deterrent to insect attack. These foods are best kept in either metal or plastic bins with close-fitting lids and which are set on roller bases for easy movement. Aluminium containers have the advantage of being both rust-proof and light weight.

Where smaller paper, polythene or plastic packages are used and where the turnover is relatively quick, it may be preferable to leave the food in those containers. These should be placed on a tray or in a shallow bin to prevent any spillage affecting food stored below.

Certain foods, such as vegetables, will need to be kept in a well-ventilated container which will hold any dirt or other debris that may become detached. These should be stored at floor level in either plastic or metal trays with perforated sides.

No container should be stored directly on the floor. Unless they are containers with roller bases, they should be put on either metal or sealed wooden duck-boards to ensure adequate circulation of air underneath.

Chilling rooms

Certain foods which do not need to be stored in a refrigerator, yet which may deteriorate more rapidly at atmospheric temperature, may be stored in a chilling room where the temperature is maintained at 3-4°C (37-39°F).

The temperature is achieved by using a chilling unit which consists of a small refrigeration unit and a fan which circulates the cold air. It is important that the unit is sufficient to maintain the low temperatures while the fan must be large enough to provide a steady but constant

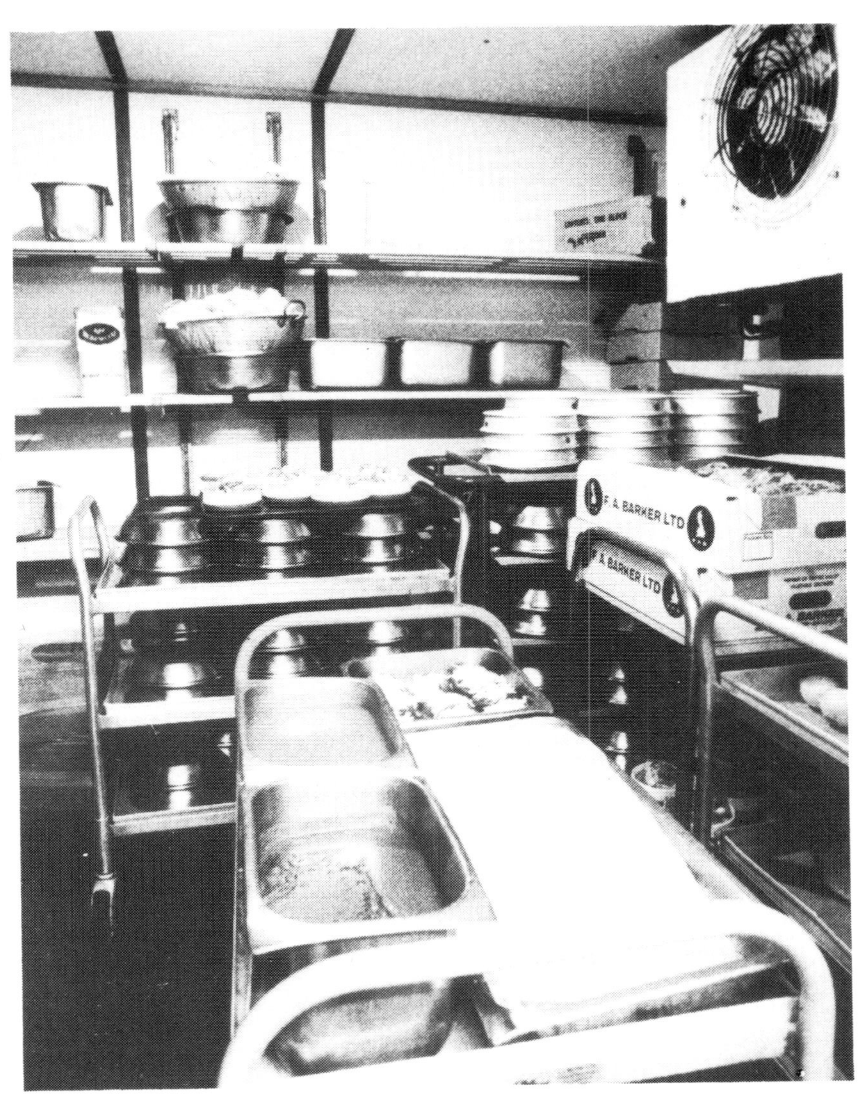

Chilling room

movement of the cold air around the food.

The same constructional details apply as for the dry store (above), except that the walls, ceiling and door should be insulated to maintain the lower temperatures.

Vegetables and milk should be kept in the chilling room. It may also be used as a preliminary store for foods which are being cooled prior to being placed in the refrigerator.

Hot food should not be placed in the refrigerator because of its effect in raising the temperature. Food which has been cooked but is not intended for immediate use, should be cooled as quickly as possible rather than be left at room temperature which would encourage bacteria to multiply. This is especially important with the so-called "danger foods", that is gravy, meat, fish and milk dishes. If allowed to cool slowly at room temperature, the bacteria within the food will multiply rapidly and, although it may be placed ultimately in the refrigerator when cool, the bacteria will merely lie dormant until the food is taken out for use.

The rule therefore for cooked food and particularly any of the "danger foods" is to place it in a chilling room as soon as possible where the temperature will be reduced quickly. As soon as the chilling temperature has been reached, it can be transferred to a refrigerator for longer periods of storage.

There may be food premises where it is not possible to provide a special chilling room, in which case a cooler part of the premises may be adapted, provided there is no risk of contamination. Although a cooling unit is only practicable in a specially-designed room, some cooling effect may be achieved merely by using a fan which itself induces a lower temperature through creating a movement of air about the food. In such cases the food should be adequately covered and should be moved into the refrigerator once the excess heat has been lost.

Cold Storage-Refrigeration

Few food premises — and certainly no catering establishment — can operate without adequate refrigeration facilities for storing food. We know that bacterial growth is reduced with any lowering of temperature and it follows that, if the temperature of food is lowered, it will not only extend its life, but will also keep it safer.

The extent to which bacterial growth is controlled will depend on the temperature. Refrigeration can preserve for days and weeks, but deep-freezing at sufficiently low temperatures can preserve for months or, in some cases, years. Readers may be aware of the food stores which had been abandoned by early explorers that have been discovered in remote parts of the world and which have remained edible through being stored at sub-zero temperatures.

Refrigeration space in the catering premises should be readily accessible and adequate in capacity. Larger premises may need the more substantial walk-in type of refrigerator, while others may rely on small commercial, or even large domestic models. In each case the temperature must be maintained at between 1-5°C (33-40°F).

Although refrigerators should be readily accessible, they should not be positioned near any source of heat. Ideally they should be in well-ventilated areas, away from the direct rays of the sun, and, if small models, should be capable of easy removal to facilitate cleaning of the surrounding area.

Construction

The larger type of walk-in refrigerator should be constructed to allow easy cleaning. When installed against walls, it should be so positioned to avoid hidden spaces which could provide a harbourage for insects and other pests. Although motors may be positioned on top of the unit, they may create noise and collect dust and are best positioned outside the main building in a properly constructed weather- and noise-proofed housing. Motors generate considerable heat in maintaining low temperatures, particularly in hot weather, and they should always be well ventilated.

Refrigerator construction usually consists of a wooden or metal exterior and a metal or plastic-coated inner skin with an insulation layer in between. The inner skin should be stainless or certainly rust-proof and shelving should likewise be of rust-proof metal on easily removable brackets.

Where existing wooden shelves are used, and assuming that they are in good condition, they should be thoroughly cleaned and scrubbed, soaked in hypochlorite solution, dried and then painted with at least two coats of polyurethane varnish to form an effective seal.

Floors should be tiled or granolithic type and should be coved to the walls for easy cleaning.

Doors will generally have a heavy rubber gasket to act as a seal. In time this can become perished and difficult to clean, so these should be checked regularly.

Smaller refrigerators are usually of all steel/enamelled metal construction and are more better designed these days so as to avoid hidden corners which can harbour dirt.

Defrosting

All refrigerators need to be serviced regularly, and defrosted strictly in accordance with the manufacturer's instructions. Failure to do so will result in a build-up of the ice layer which will lower the efficiency of the unit. Also the motor has to work unnecessarily hard to maintain the temperature, which of course rapidly increases the electricity consumption.

When refrigerators are defrosted, all surfaces should be thoroughly cleaned at the same time. This includes the removal and cleaning of shelving and duck boards. If it is intended to close down the refrigerator, it should be defrosted, cleaned and thoroughly dried to prevent any mould formation. Ideally, doors should be left open slightly to encourage a constant circulation of air.

When it is intended to defrost a refrigerator, the contents should be run down as far as possible and any remaining food should either be placed in another refrigerator, or be covered and stored in a cool place, or wrapped in several layers of clean paper to contain as much of the coldness as possible.

Using the refrigerator

The storage within a refrigerator is important and certain rules should be observed. It should not be overcrowded, otherwise it is not possible to maintain the necessary circulation of air. All food should be adequately covered and under no circumstances should raw foods — especially raw meat — be allowed to come into contact with other food. The reason is the danger of contamination from the raw food to that food which may be consumed without any further cooking. Besides protecting the food from contamination, adequate covering will also help prevent any drying out or possible absorption of odour from certain foods.

Hot food should never be placed in the refrigerator because it raises the temperature and the steam can cause a build-up of ice on the cooling unit. Those foods which tend to be wet or moist, should be kept in suitable trays or other containers to prevent dripping. Tin foil or one of the many cellophane wrapping materials now available provide an excellent covering for most types of food.

Although foods will keep very well in a refrigerator at the correct temperature for many days, the longer they are kept the more likelihood there will be of some loss of quality. When stacking a refrigerator with a fresh delivery, it is very important to bring old stock to the front so that it will be used first.

Freezers

Whilst chilling and refrigeration temperatures represent levels at which foods may be stored, an extension whereby even lower temperatures are involved is found in deep freezer storage. The temperature here is around -18°C (0°F), and has the effect of killing off many organisms, including some of those in the *Salmonella* group, and greatly retarding bacterial growth generally.

As with refrigerators, food must not be packed in freezers so tight that a circulation of cold air cannot be maintained.

Freezing is intended to keep sound food longer and manufacturers take great care to ensure that only sound food is processed initially. Various methods of freezing foods exist including liquid nitrogen, blast freezing and plate freezing designed to "quick freeze". These techniques have been developed to reduce enzyme activity, destroy bacterial cells and prevent destruction of the food cells so that the nutritional value (vitamins) and quality are maintained on thawing.

Deep freezers should be defrosted and cleaned regularly and the food itself should be examined periodically to check on damage to both itself and to wrappings. Stock rotation is essential as even frozen food has a "shelf life". Deliveries of frozen food should be transferred to the freezer immediately on receipt.

Many catering establishments use open-top freezers similar to those found in supermarkets and stores. Although the same rules for cleanliness and stacking apply as for all refrigerators, it is essential here to ensure that food is not placed above the load line. This is a red line usually marked on the sides of the cabinet, below which freezer temperatures are maintained, yet above which the temperature rises rapidly. If, therefore, the food is stored above the load line it becomes subject to these higher temperatures, which can seriously affect the quality.

Deep frozen food

Frozen food should be used within the time recommended by the manufacturer. As a rule, foods that have thawed should not be re-frozen because this will cause cell structure damage, loss of colour, nutritional value and quality. Food which has been refrozen and subsequently thoroughly cooked is quite safe, but the flavour and texture will be below the high quality of quick-frozen foods.

The "star" rating used in connection with frozen food is intended as a guide for storage and operates as follows:

* Has a storage life of up to 1 week;

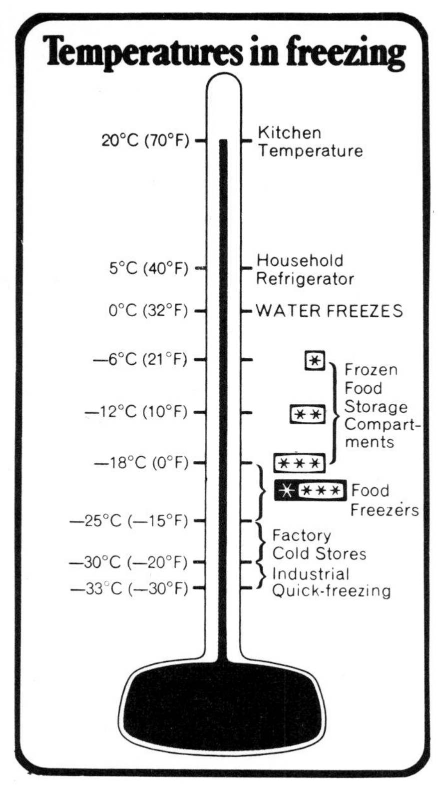

(By courtesy of Birds Eye Food Ltd)

** Has a storage life of up to 1 month;
*** Has a storage life of up to 3 months.

Ice-cream is one popular frozen food which has been marketed and developed very successfully over the years. It is a useful food to take as an example of the careful handling and storage required for frozen food. Ice-cream is one of the potentially dangerous foods, because it is an excellent medium in which bacteria can multiply. For this reason, very strict hygiene precautions are taken in the manufacture of ice-cream and temperatures are carefully monitored throughout the process and its subsequent storage. In fact, if the temperature rises above —2°C (28°F), the ice-cream must be reprocessed. While wrapped ice-cream is generally safe from contamination, there is a common practice in catering of using bulk ice-cream in polythene containers. The lids must be kept on such containers and scoops or serving utensils must be kept in a suitable disinfectant solution when not in use to prevent bacterial contamination.

Chapter 7

PEST CONTROL

To most people the presence of rats, mice, flies, cockroaches and even spiders is revolting and always associated with dirty conditions. It is for precisely these reasons that extreme care must be exercised in food premises to prevent the introduction of such pests or, alternatively, to ensure immediate steps are taken to exterminate them, once their presence is detected.

This chapter describes the various species of pest commonly encountered in Britain, the methods of control available and the preventative measures which can be used.

It cannot be overemphasised that the presence of vermin costs money and causes trouble for the food industry. The total cost of rat and mice infestations, in terms of contaminated food and damaged buildings and equipment, runs into tens of millions of pounds each year in Britain alone.

Several species of pest present a risk to human health by carrying bacteria which survive and multiply in suitable foods, and which may subsequently be the cause of illness in the consumer.

Rats and mice

These rodents are commonly encountered in urban and rural areas alike and are recognised carriers of several diseases harmful to man. In particular, they are known sources of infection for plague, leptospirosis and food poisoning.

Rats and mice are particularly attracted to food premises because of the presence of their basic requirements: food, drink and shelter. Dirty premises, poor housekeeping and undisturbed cover are ideal.

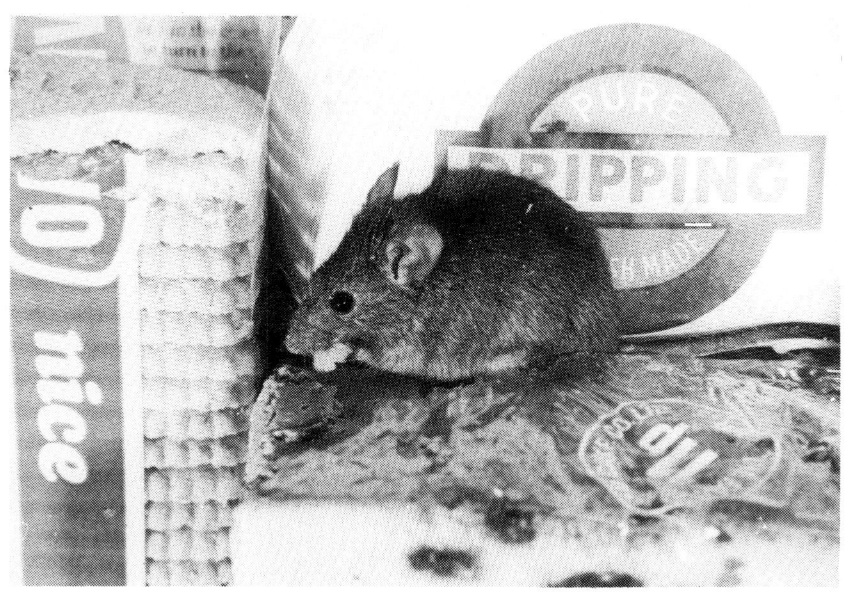

The mouse — an unwanted visitor in food premises (Rentokil Ltd)

The common or brown rat is the species most often encountered in this country, although the black or ship rat is occasionally found in dockland areas. The adult brown rat is about 25cm (10in) long, weighs 330 grams (12 oz) and has a blunt muzzle, small ears and a short stout tail. The colour of the coat varies from brown to grey.

Rats and mice are prolific breeders; the young are born in litters of between four and ten. They reach maturity in three months and the females have three or four litters a year — one pair could produce a thousand offspring a year.

The house mouse is a cross between tame and field mice which produces a wide range of colour and size variations. The adult mouse is about 56mm (2¼in) long, the muzzle is pointed, it has large and furry ears and a long tail. Mice are generally more difficult to kill than rats. The presence of droppings is the surest indication of an infestation of rats or mice. Signs of damage, such as gnawing of boxes, sacks, woodwork around doors, and even damaged lead pipes are also indicative of infestation, as are smear marks around pipes and walls.

While it is possible to eradicate a rat or mouse infestation using do-it-yourself techniques such as trapping and even poisoning, such methods are not really recommended for the food trade. Firstly there are definite techniques and "tricks of the trade" which the amateur would not know; and secondly few people would have the time to devote to ensuring that the rodents were destroyed quickly and efficiently. It is therefore suggested that the local Council's Environmental Health Department or a private pest control firm be employed to eradicate the pests. It is also worth considering engaging a contractor to inspect and treat the premises regularly, but this aspect is dealt with more fully later in the chapter.

Cats are often thought to be a good deterrent and may even catch an odd rat or mouse, but domestic pets should not be encouraged in food premises as they may harbour various diseases and parasites themselves. Cats are not therefore recommended.

Flies

These are probably the commonest insect pest found in food premises, and the dirtiest. There are over 3,000 different species of flies found in Britain and over 50,000 different species in the world. Flies are a potential danger to health because they are capable of contaminating food and transmitting disease. These insects are believed to spread cholera, typhoid, dysentery, poliomyelitis and food poisoning. The house fly (*Musca domestica*), the cluster fly, the blow-fly, the blue-bottle and the

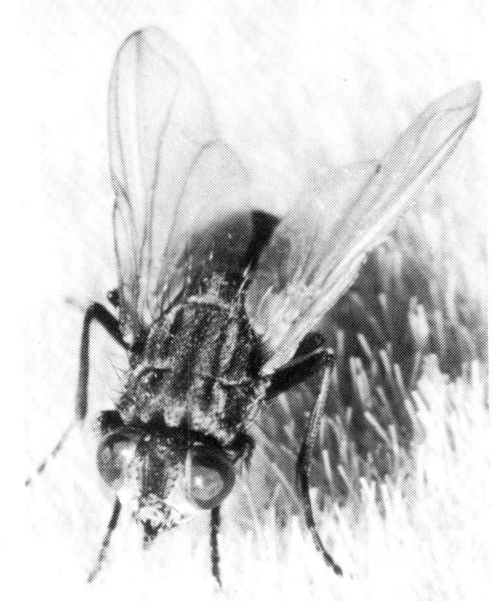

The fly — a champion germ carrier (Rentokil Ltd)

mosquito are the most important and frequent invaders of buildings.

Flies feed on a variety of rejected foods, refuse and the excrement of man and animals. They will feed on food, contaminate it and lay eggs on it at the same time. Many contaminated foods will be eaten without further cooking and this is why every effort should be made to exterminate flies. The most effective way of controlling flies is to prevent them breeding by efficient refuse storage, elimination of compost heaps, removal of similar accumulations, and the storage of food in fly-proof containers.

Flies will multiply at an alarming rate; one female lays 100-150 eggs which will hatch and develop into adults in 7 to 14 days, depending on weather conditions.

Windows can be fitted with fine mesh screens, and hanging strips of plastic can be placed across doorways effectively.

Aerosol fly-sprays can be used inside buildings, although not in food rooms. Flypaper strips are being reintroduced and insecticide lacquers can be applied to wall surfaces to provide methods of destroying flies. The installation of an ultra-violet light electrocutor can be very effective and certainly overcomes the old problem of dead insects falling into the food!

Cockroaches

These insects are frequently encountered in food premises of all types, from bakeries to cafes and hotels to hospitals. Like flies, these thrive in greasy, wet, dirty, warm conditions. The adults are large ugly insects whose main danger is their ability to carry disease organisms, particularly food poisoning bacteria, which can contaminate food and equipment. Cockroaches are nocturnal insects, so that an infestation can build up undetected unless the premises are used at night when there is more likelihood of the insects being seen.

There are two species of cockroach commonly found in Britain, namely the German cockroach (*Blatella germanica*), familiarly known as the "steam fly", and the Oriental (or common) cockroach (*Blatta orientalis*), also known as the black beetle, The Oriental cockroach is twice as long as the German cockroach. These insects favour inaccessible places, such as pipe ducts, lift shafts, bases of fixed ovens and cupboards, and lay their eggs in capsules out of reach of insecticides. This is why infestations cannot be immediately eradicated other than by a carefully phased programme of treatments, plus associated building maintenance works to deal with structural faults.

Strict attention to hygiene is essential to prevent food supplies being available to the insects while the efficient design, construction and

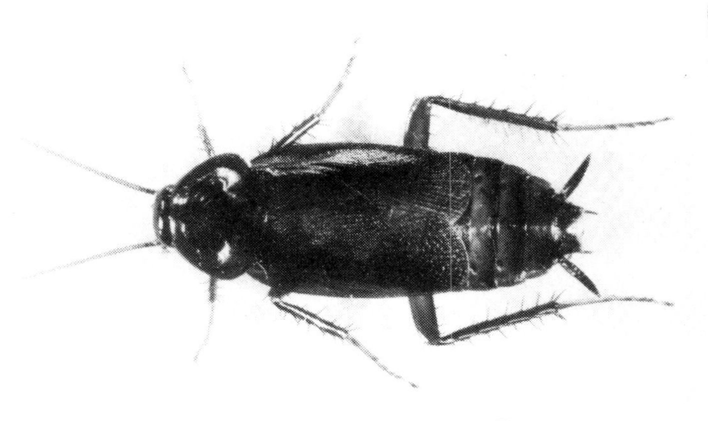

The cockroach — another enemy of the caterer (Rentokil Ltd)

maintenance of buildings and equipment will reduce the possibility of infestations occurring or being allowed to build up.

Dealing with an infestation is best left to trained staff from a commercial pest control company or a local authority. Various techniques can be used to eradicate the pests. The most effective treatment combines a pyrethrum-based insecticide to kill the young nymphs and adult insects, with a residual insecticide in the form of a lacquer sprayed or painted around the likely breeding places. The search for new and effective insecticides continues because cockroaches are particularly adept at producing an immunity or resistance to particular chemicals after a while.

Ants

These insects frequently invade food premises and domestic dwellings in search of food, particularly sugar-based products. Colonies of ants, particularly the black garden ant (*Lasius niger*), are found in gardens or under paved areas; the much smaller Pharaoh's ant [*Monomorium pharaonis*) breeds in the fabric of a building, around catering equipment and heating duct pipes. The garden ant can be dealt with by tracing and destroying the nest. However the Pharaoh's ant is more difficult to eradicate and needs a thorough investigation and treatment by a competent operator.

Wasps

Another insect attracted to food premises in its search for sugar-based food, fruit and beer, they are principally a nuisance. They are only a danger to human beings who may be allergic to a wasp sting. Adult insects can be prevented from gaining access to a building by fitting fly-proof screening to doors and windows. Insecticide strips may be used or preferably ultra-violet light electrocutor units can attract and kill the insects. The destruction of wasps' nests can be undertaken by purchasing a quantity of a proprietary powder and carefully following the instructions; or by employing the services of a commercial pest control company or the local authority, if it operates such a service to commerce.

Pests in stored products

Many insect pests attack not only growing crops but also stored food products in factories, warehouses and larders. A small selection of the common insects would include:

Book lice	Insects infest flour and cereals
Biscuit beetle	Grubs attack cereals, biscuits and flour
Cheese & ham skipper	A maggot or larva infesting decomposing meat, ham, bacon or over-ripe cheese
Drug-store beetle	Bread and some drugs
Flour beetles	Insects feeding on flour or broken cereals
Flour moth & Warehouse moth	Attack flour, milled cereals, dried fruits, chocolate, spices and nuts
Grain & rice weevils	Attack any whole grain
Larder beetle	Attacks most foods and materials of an animal origin
Mites	Very small insects, almost "dust", which infest stored and packaged foods
Spider beetles	The grubs or larvae will feed on almost any food, carpets and clothing

Preventative measures include the frequent examination and rotation of food stocks. Once an infestation has been discovered it is essential to remove the foodstuffs and have them destroyed, while the premises can be disinfested using a suitable insecticide. It is recommended that the advice of the local Environmental Health Officer is obtained on the correct treatment.

Birds

Various species of birds have become an increasing problem in recent years. Apart from the damage and defacement they cause to buildings, their nests and droppings can present a serious risk to health. Pigeons, for example, are known to transmit *Salmonella* organisms. Starlings, sparrows, even finches and bluetits have become unwelcome invaders of food factories. Preventative measures include netting and sealing of access points, and the provision of gelatenous material along parapets and walls to prevent birds from perching or nesting on these surfaces.

Eradication measures usually involve extermination by narcotic poisoning, or shooting using high-powered air rifles. Once again, these measures should be left to experienced pest control companies.

Control measures

As already indicated, there are three methods of eradicating vermin and pests from premises: namely

1. do-it-yourself;
2. commercial pest control companies;
3. the local authority Pest Control service.

Undertaking the destruction of an infestation by an amateur has the principle attraction of appearing to save money. Many chemists, ironmongers and garden-supplies shops stock entire ranges of insecticides and rodenticides, such as Warfarin and alphachlorolose.

By carefully following the instructions, it is possible successfully to deal with an invasion of mice, flies, ants — even cockroaches and rats. Mousetraps can also be effectually used if flour, sugar or chocolate is placed on the spike instead of cheese, the balance finely set and the trap placed at right angles against the wall. Insects can be controlled with the use of aerosol insecticide sprays, provided care is taken not to use them where food is liable to contamination. The same warning applies to the use of hanging blocks or strips of material which emit a gradual quantity of insecticide over a period of months. The authors understand that the "old fashioned" sticky flypaper is being re-marketed successfully as a safer alternative.

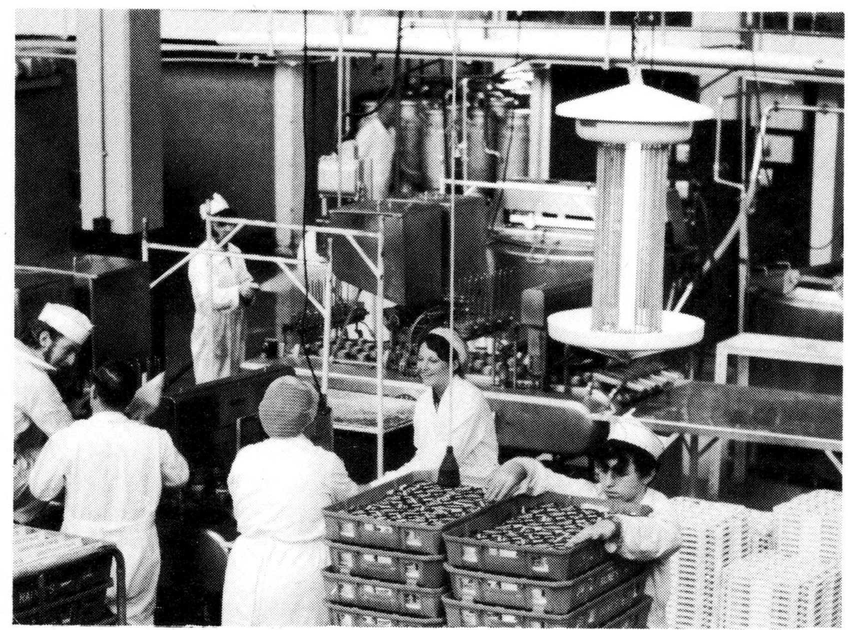

An ultra-violet electric insect-killer in a food factory (Rentokil Ltd)

Although not strictly a do-it-yourself measure, the purchase or hiring of an ultra-violet light insect "killer" apparatus does involve the regular cleaning of the lower tray and the renewal of the strip light from year to year because of the gradual reduction in the effectiveness of the light as an attraction for the insects. Incidentally these units operate most efficiently at night, when insects such as wasps are least active. Nevertheless the installation of one or more in a food room will reduce the flying insect population and thereby the risk of contamination; even the "fly in the soup" will be less of a possibility.

All reputable pest control servicing companies belong to the British Pest Control Association and membership of that association is a reliable guide to the quality of the contractor. The major commercial companies have built up a reputation over many years, have extensive laboratory facilities and well-trained staff. Most contractors offer a service based on a simple treatment to remove the current pest infestation and/or a contract to call at specified intervals to survey and carry out any necessary treatment for certain pests or any species of pest.

Many local authorities offer a similar service to commerce and industry through their Environmental Health Department and trained staff are employed to deal with most types of vermin and pests. Inquiries should be made to the Council Offices, because some authorities prefer to leave pest control in food premises to the commercial companies; the principal reason being to avoid any conflict of interest arising with the Council's legal responsibilities to enforce the legislation in those premises.

It should be emphasised that if a contractor is employed, and especially if a contract is signed for pest control work to be undertaken, this does not absolve or indemnify the owner or proprietor of a food business from his responsibilities under the Food Hygiene Regulations to "keep the premises free from infestation by vermin or insect pests". Few contractors call regularly enough to give an effective "guarantee" against infestation and the costs associated with, say, a weekly survey would be too prohibitive for most businesses.

It is therefore essential that persons responsible for food premises should keep a constant watch for signs of pest infestations, keep the premises in a clean and tidy condition inside and out, and maintain a cleaning standard which is linked to stock rotation and the prevention of food and refuse accumulating.

Preventative measures

It is also possible to take certain preventative measures to reduce the risk of infestations occurring. These include erecting fly screens to open windows during the summer months; placing fine mesh behind air bricks and metal plates at the bottom of external doors and frames to stop vermin from gnawing through the wood; replacing wooden floors and skirting with concrete; keeping refuse bins off the ground; ensuring that there are no sources of water for pests to drink; sealing holes and gaps around pipes, drains and other openings in walls and floors; fixing tiles and wall coverings directly onto brick or plastered walls, not battening, which provides a cavity; and keeping the building in good repair.

Although unsightly it is better to leave pipes unlagged or encased in ducting than provide possible harbourage for insects to live and breed. Special attention should be paid to any lift-shafts in the building, because these are favourite sites for infestations.

All food supplies should be kept in vermin-proof containers, preferably metal, although it is accepted that this is not always practicable. Cases of food should not be stacked against walls or into corners. The practice of painting floor/wall junctions with white paint encourages cleanliness and makes a new infestation easier to spot.

Stock rotation is of vital importance, both from a food freshness and an infestation control angle. Attention to cleanliness, especially removing spillage in food rooms, will reduce the food supply and the attraction for the insect or rodent.

Chapter 8

PERSONAL HEALTH AND HYGIENE

Some people go through life without having a day off work through illness and are rightly proud of this achievement; other people seem prone to illness and are forever calling the doctor. Undoubtedly there are reasons why the viruses and bacteria which cause disease attack the weak person, and this is largely due to the poor resistance which such a body's defence mechanisms can put up against a massive invasion of these foreign bodies. The first line of defence is our skin. The second line of defence is the white blood cells (leucocytes) whose job is to isolate foreign bodies in the blood and kill them if possible. The third defensive system is the lymph ducts and glands which act as filters to stop bacteria spreading round the body, and finally there are the liver and spleen to act as further filters for the blood and digestive system. These defensive systems can be weakened by a general lowering of a person's health due to the stress and strain of modern living. This can be either physical, due to lack of sleep or overwork, or mental, due to worry over personal or family problems.
over personal or family problems.

There are a large number of contagious or infectious diseases. Some of them are common childhood diseases, such as measles or whooping cough. Others cause severe illness, even death, such as poliomyelitis, meningitis and typhoid. Most people know that these diseases are spread from infectious persons, either by direct contact or contamination, or by droplet infection through sneezing or just breathing in the virus causing the disease. There are even people who have suffered from a disease, apparently recovered and, unbeknown to them, have retained a reservoir of infection in their bodies. Subsequently they become "healthy carriers", continually but innocently infecting other persons. Knowledge of these ways of spreading diseases is particularly important when dealing with food hygiene because so many foods are ideal material on which the bacteria can survive and multiply, and therefore personal health and hygiene are vitally important.

Let us examine the most important diseases associated with food:

Dysentery and Diarrhoea are particularly prevalent in schools and large institutions where poor cloakroom hygiene, shared equipment and toys are all links in the chain.

Typhoid and Paratyphoid are waterborne diseases which are rare in Britain, although endemic in some countries, due largely to the lack of adequate sewerage and water purification systems.

Dermatitis is probably the most common industrial disease causing lengthy absences. Yet it is largely preventable. Bacterial or fungal infections are usually to blame, aggravated by handling chemicals or other materials (such as flour or sugar) or just by friction from continual handling of commodities.

Food Poisoning is, of course, the subject of a separate chapter in this book and is perhaps the disease most closely associated with food, as the name implies.

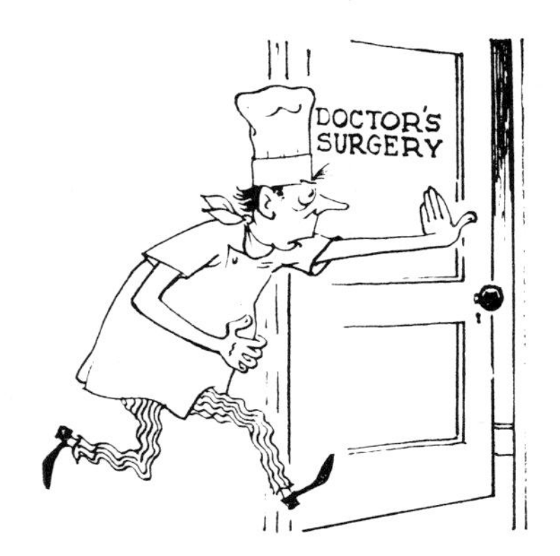

With the exception of dermatitis, all the other diseases mentioned above, together with a further twenty five, are notifiable infectious diseases. This means that they have to be notified to the local authority by the doctor who is treating the patient. In addition, under the provisions of the Food Hygiene Regulations, if a food handler becomes aware that he is suffering from one of the infectious diseases listed, then he must notify the person carrying on the food business who must then notify the local authority. In this way the risk of infected food being sold to the public is minimised, but a big responsibility rests on the individual food handlers, be they in a factory or a home.

Most large food manufacturing companies take a special interest in the health and welfare of their staff; indeed, they have a statutory responsibility to do so under the Health & Safety at Work Act, 1974. Typically each prospective employee is asked to complete a medical history of previous illnesses, followed by a detailed medical examination, which includes submitting a faecal specimen for laboratory examination. The authors understand that a surprisingly large number of applicants are rejected because of poor health and personal hygiene: ear infections, septic skins, boils, dirty bodies, nits, carious teeth, bad hands, marked obesity, bronchitis, osteoarthritis, dyspepsia and severe varicose veins are some of the more common reasons. Some of these symptoms can be remedied quite easily and frequently the applicants return much improved, and are able to maintain their healthier condition when subsequently employed. This lack of interest or concern for one's personal health and hygiene is a sad reflection on the education system, which apparently fails to emphasise the basic necessities of a healthy life.

Personal hygiene

Whenever or wherever food is handled, whether in the shop, restaurant, factory or the home, one of the most critical factors is the personal hygiene of the handler. The main criterion is that any person who is suffering from any disease mentioned in the preceding paragraphs, or from attacks of diarrhoea or vomiting, skin infections, boils or infected wounds, discharging ears or nose and throat infections should avoid handling food or utensils. Even healthy people carry some germs in the nose, throat, bowel and on the skin.

The mouth, nose and particularly the hands, are the most critical areas of the human body because these are the organs where germs can harbour, multiply and subsequently contaminate food and materials. In the "old days", young people were taught the basic rules of hygiene by their parents and school teachers, but, as the modern generations do not appear to receive this type of education, it might be useful to review these rules and the reasons for them:

1. Wash your hands thoroughly before starting work, after handling

raw foods, frequently whilst handling different foods, and after visiting the lavatory. Reasons — see the special section on hand-washing.
2. Keep fingernails short and clean; do not use nail varnish.
Reasons – because fingernails harbour dirt and bacteria, also nail varnish can chip off into the food.
3. Keep cuts or burns covered with waterproof dressings.
Reason — to prevent cuts being infected which makes them slow to heal. It also enables the hands to be washed without the dressing becoming wet and useless and prevents the food from being contaminated by septic matter from the wound.
4. Do not smoke or take snuff when handling food.
Reasons — apart from the proven danger to health from smoking, the main risks are that these habits entail the hands being in contact with the nose and/or mouth and consequently the fingers can transfer nose and throat infections (especially *Staphylococcus*).
5. Do not lick fingers when handling food or wrapping materials.
Reasons — as for smoking.
6. Do not pick your nose, teeth or ears, or scratch your backside.
Reasons – various infections and bacteria can be resident in these locations and the fingers will act as the vehicle for spread of infection to other persons, materials and food in particular.
8. Do not cough or sneeze over food.
Reasons — a sneeze contains millions of bacteria which spread over a wide area by means of droplets. Contamination can best be reduced by using a paper handkerchief.
9. Do not scratch your head.
Reasons — the scalp can be both dirty due to atmospheric contamination and full of infection such as dandruff, which is transferred to the fingernails and subsequently to food.
Hair should be completely covered when handling food. This applies to men and women alike; no-one likes to find hairs in their food — even clean ones!
10. Do not use an overall, apron or cloth to wipe the hands.
Reasons — these habits only spread bacteria and give rise to bigger risks as the bacteria or dirt accumulates. Hand-washing is the only acceptable method of keeping hands clean.

Handling Food

"Food should be handled as little as possible." This is a golden rule of hygiene but is easier said than done. There is no doubt that many

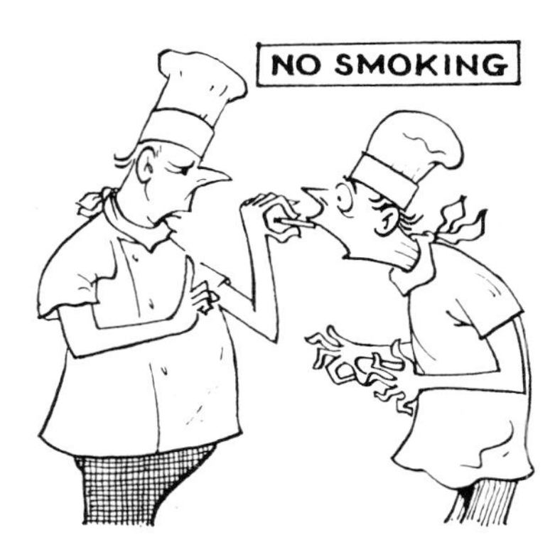

outbreaks of food poisoning can be traced to bad practices which involve unnecessary handling of food. A particular danger is the practice of handling raw food, and then handling cooked or semi-cooked food without stopping to cleanse the hands and equipment in between. Poultry, meat products and pet foods are particularly prone to *Salmonella* infection and these bacteria, counted in millions, will be transferred to other foods by cross-contamination, with dire consequences.

If possible, food should be "handled" by clean utensils such as tongs which are to be found in most baker's and grocer's shops. Hygiene is a way of life, and it is a good habit which will be appreciated by friends and customers the world over. Of course, there are many facets of food preparation and cooking where handling is unavoidable, and this is where clean hands and forearms are vitally important.

Cleaning the hands

Hand-washing should be a very frequent habit when handling food. A washhand basin with hot and cold running water, bactericidal soap, nail brush and a paper towel dispenser or hot air dryer should be standard equipment fitted conveniently close to all preparation areas. Washhand basins should be kept exclusively for the purpose and not used as small sinks for utensils or vegetable washing. Likewise sinks should not be used for hand-washing because the tendency is to "rinse" the hands under the tap (cold or scalding hot) with dangerous and most unsatisfactory results.

Hand-washing must be thorough, using plenty of hot soapy water and a nailbrush to scrub the skin and the fingernails.

Remember that some bacteria will resist removal after five minutes' hand-washing, which is why bactericidal soaps and creams have been introduced. Heat alone will not kill some germs but the chemical sterilants will do so.

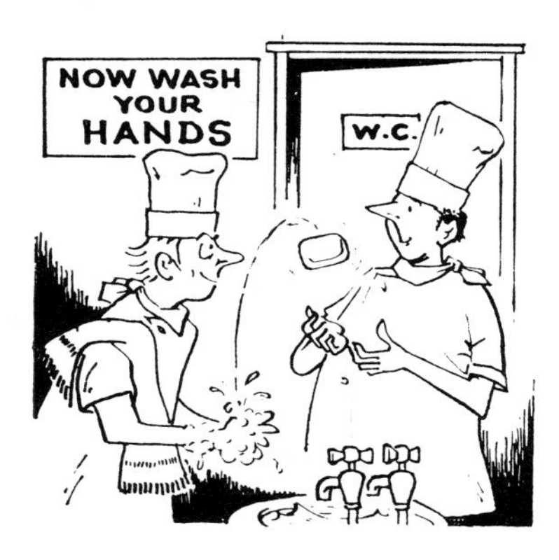

It is no use washing the hands thoroughly and then drying them on an ordinary towel or roller towel, because you will probably recontaminate your hands with the previous person's germs. Disposable paper towels or warm air dryers are the answer, as are elbow-operated taps or foot operated taps over washhand basins if one is going to be truly clinical about avoiding cross-contamination.

Most people are taught to wash their hands after using the toilet, but how many people only rinse their fingers under the cold tap as a token gesture? The human bowel carries millions of bacteria, most of which are essential to the body, but a few species of which are disease-causing organisms. Failure to observe this elementary rule exposes other people to infection, which can be picked up on the lavatory seat, chain or lever, door handle, tap, towels and light switch.

Hand cleansers and hand drying

Soap itself can harbour germs and experiments have shown that many soaps are ineffective in removing bacteria; their main value is in dissolving grease and surface dirt. For this reason the installation of a liquid or gel-type soap (containing hexachlorophane or a similar bacteria killer) dispenser at each washhand basin is recommended.

Hand creams are available to act as cleansers where soiled hands need deep cleansing prior to washing, and as barrier creams after hand-washing to protect the skin against irritants such as salts and chemicals. The use of thin polythene transparent disposable gloves may be an alternative solution in certain circumstances.

The old fashioned roller towel is not acceptable because it means that people, after a while, begin to use the same piece of towel. Automatic roller towel cabinets are better although the mechanism can sometimes stick and one has to make sure that replacement towels are readily available. It should be noted that few laundries operate a towel cleaning service which is completely acceptable in terms of bacterial condition.

Paper towels are commonly used today and provide a complete answer to the objections just mentioned as each person uses a separate dry clean towel. Regular removal of the waste paper should not be overlooked. Electrical hot air hand dryers are usually foot operated and are found to be successful except in the event of a power cut or breakdown; an emergency supply of paper towels is the obvious reserve. The authors have not attempted a cost benefit analysis of the two recommended methods because of the escalating costs of electricity and paper respectively.

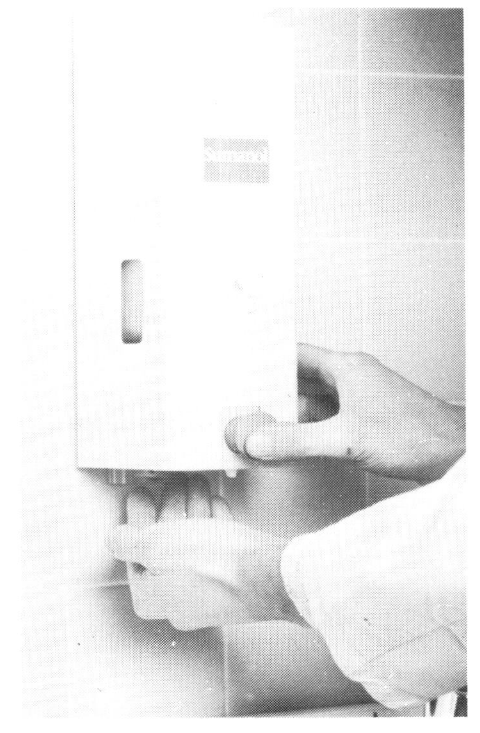

Bactericidal soap dispenser (Lever Industrial Ltd)

Sanitary accommodation
Lavatories are an essential feature of modern living, but how many people appreciate the potential hazard to health which they present? As previously mentioned, the human intestine contains quantities of harmful and harmless bacteria. These harmful bacteria may not affect the carrier but can be spread to other people by carelessness, bad habits and the water closet. The first two causes have been explained, but did you realise that even with the seat and lid closed the flushing of the W.C. spreads germs into the air, on to the seat, the floor, and under the flushing rim of the pan. Dysentery bacteria can live up to four weeks in faecal matter. The thorough cleansing and disinfection of lavatories and associated apparatus is essential if they are to cease to convey disease-causing organisms.

Many people, especially women, have a justifiable aversion to using public or communal lavatories because of their fear of catching diseases, such as dysentery. This disdain is well founded because of the generally poor standard of hygiene, maintenance and furnishing of sanitary conveniences in this country. It is a sad reflection, however, that it is the users who create the unsavoury conditions in the first instance. In food premises, only the highest standards of equipment and maintenance should be provided in order to reduce the risk of spread of disease to an absolute minimum. Special attention should be given to frequent cleansing of fittings, handles, walls, floors and doors with disinfectants, the provision of pilfer-proof toilet-roll holders and their replenishment.

The cloakroom should be well lighted and ventilated in accordance with the minimum standards required by the Building Regulations, 1976, the Food Hygiene Regulations, 1970, and the Health & Safety at Work Act, 1974. The sanitary accommodation provided for females should be fitted with an incinerator or a sanitary dressing disposal unit which is regularly serviced by one of the commercial hygiene companies now operating in the country. This is a legal requirement wherever several females are employed.

Animals
Under no circumstances should pet animals be allowed access to food preparation rooms. Cats and dogs carry a number of diseases transmissible to man, including the *Toxicaria* round-worm.

Cats are particularly prone to jumping onto preparation tables, and their paws will distribute germs whilst their moulting coats will leave a trail of hairs. Hand-washing after handling a pet animal is vital, and similarly ensuring that no animal is allowed to eat from a dish or container normally used for human food, or vice versa! Utensils and equipment, such as knives, cutting boards and saucepans should be used exclusively for animal food. Animal food stored in the refrigerator should ideally be double-wrapped.

Protective clothing

The Food Hygiene Regulations refer to "persons handling open food to wear over-clothing", etc and state that any person who engages in the handling of open food must wear sufficient clean and washable over-clothing. The purpose is two-fold. Firstly, and more important, a person's everyday clothing may become soiled and in the course of preparation may come into contact with the food. We all know how easily clothes may become soiled and in addition to basic dirt and dust, clothes may become soiled by animals who have been in close contact.

The second reason is to protect the worker himself from soiling his own clothes by the food which could then give rise to cross-contamination.

The Regulations require 'sufficient' clean over-clothing, which means that it must adequately cover the person to the extent of covering any part of the person's body that may come into contact with the food or equipment. It must also be clean. In the past there has been much argument over what is clean. Bearing in mind that an excellent definition of clean is an absence of dirt, you might assume that any over-clothing, however slightly soiled, should be changed. Clearly, this is intended to be interpreted sensibly and what it seeks to prevent is a coat or apron which is so soiled that it is a real source of contamination as opposed to one which has a small amount of dirt, which one must accept with the handling process.

A butcher is most likely to require a clean apron every day, whilst a grocer may only need one every two days. It is a question of degree and generalisations are dangerous.

Although the need to wear suitable over-clothing applies to most food handlers there are exceptions for those who are only handling raw vegetables, intoxicating liquor or soft drinks. This means that a person working behind a bar in a pub need not wear over-clothing, *although* it does mean that once food is handled over-clothing is necessary.

This is an aspect of the Food Hygiene Regulations which is often overlooked especially by publicans. One reason for this is that the traditional role of the publican has changed considerably since the original Regulations were introduced, to the extent that now the service of

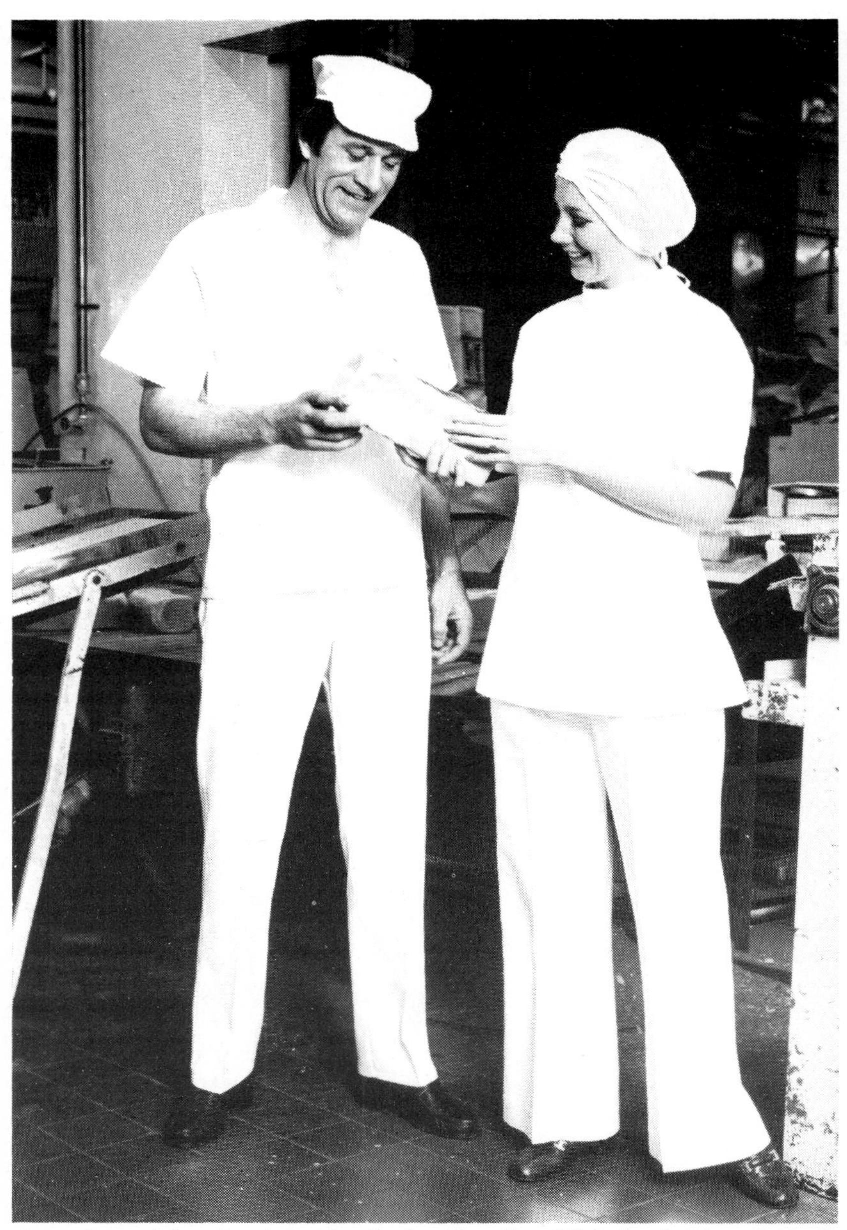

Attractive and functional clothing for food handlers (Nicholson's (Overalls) Ltd)

food has become a substantial part of the public house trade, especially at mid-day. While few local authorities are likely to take it literally, it is none the less left to the Environmental Health Officer's discretion as to whether he insists upon suitable over-clothing where food is handled. Most authorities tend not to ask for any over-clothing though there is an increasing number who do where the handling of food behind the bar is substantial.

The choice of over-clothing is important and light colours are preferable as they show up any dirt more readily. Many employers justifiably regard clean over-clothing as a psychological boost to staff. In the United States a report was issued a few years ago which stated that employers who made an ample supply of clean coats available to their staff were rewarded very often by them taking more pride in themselves and in their work which, of course, resulted in a better work performance. This practice has been copied by most of the more hygiene conscious firms in the United Kingdom. Any company policy to make clean coats available as and when necessary (as opposed to only once every two, three or so many days) clearly is desirable and should be encouraged.

Modern materials do not restrict employees to the rather clinical heavy cotton coats once available in "all shades of white". Modern colours as well as designs are available and have much more appeal especially to the fashion-conscious female personnel. Drip-dry fabrics tend not to absorb or retain dirt and can, of course, be laundered much more easily.

In recent years disposable aprons have been introduced which act as an outer protection to the normal over-clothing and which are especially useful where more dirty tasks are involved such as washing up or dressing poultry. In any case, an outer rubberised or plastic apron is useful where water is involved. Aprons should also be available so that even though a handler may not normally be involved with a dirty process he should be able to put one on rather than risk dirtying his main over-clothing.

The need for hair covering has caused much argument over the years and more especially with younger female (and not always female!) staff who object to having to bundle their hair together. The purpose of hair covering is principally three-fold. Firstly, and from the food hygiene point of view, it is intended to keep hair out of the food. Secondly, it helps to keep hair dry and free from grease in a kitchen and, thirdly, and this applies to safety, keeps the hair from becoming tangled in any machinery such as mixers and grinders.

As with other over-clothing modern designs have made them far more acceptable to staff and they range from the traditional cotton cook's hat to the turban type muslin mesh headscarves which tend to be more suitable for female personnel. What is important is that all the long hair and, indeed, most of the hair itself is covered. Needless to say, hair should never be combed in a food room.

The choice of footwear is also important though often overlooked. While shoes are unlikely to come into contact with the food, they are none the less part of over-clothing and should be kept clean. They should also be practical in that they provide a safe footing for those who may be working on slippery surfaces or who are expected to climb stairs or steps.

Storage arrangements for clothing is important and the Regulations are explicit in that "...subject to any certificate of exemption, there shall be provided in all food premises where open food is handled suitable and sufficient accommodation for out-door and other clothing or footwear not being worn during working hours ... and this clothing and footwear shall only be kept in accommodation specially provided . . ." Where no special provision is made outside the food room such clothing may only be kept in the food room if in suitable lockers or cupboards.

In most food premises a separate room is set aside, perhaps as a staff room, where mackintoshes, coats and so on may be hung. Where this is not available then a suitable locker or cupboard must be provided which allows for the clothing to be hung and which can be closed. The provision of a staff room or similar is preferable as, if outdoor clothing is wet, it has a better chance of drying than if it is hanging in the confined space of a cupboard or locker within a food room.

First aid

All food premises must provide a first aid kit which must be readily accessible to all staff. A kit kept locked in a cupboard with only one key, that is not available when the holder is away, is not acceptable. It should be kept in a staff room or at least nearby the food room so that if a person is injured he can turn to it quickly. Desirably, it should be near to a wash basin so that any injury can be washed and dressed without delay.

The containers should be suitably labelled and a member of staff should be held responsible for ensuring that it is adequately stocked. This same person should ideally have some elementary training in first aid and should be known to all the personnel. A notice indicating who this person is and where he may be contacted should be either indicated on the kit or on a notice nearby.

While the larger manufacturing and retail firms usually have a full-time nurse in charge of a sick room, most firms arrange for selected

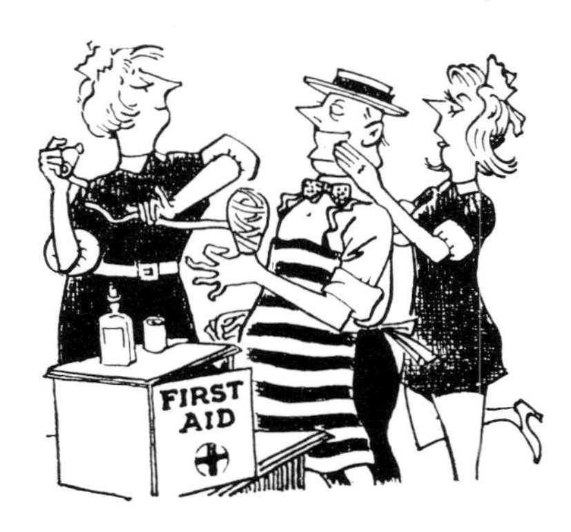

staff to undergo some training in first aid. Such courses are available in most districts and very good short courses are always available through either the British Red Cross or the St. John's Ambulance Brigade. Needless to say, a first aid box without someone to use it sensibly is useless.

The contents of the first aid box is important and it should contain "... a sufficient supply of suitable bandages, dressings (including water-proof dressings) and antiseptic ... " (Food Hygiene Regulations).

It is a good idea to use one of the coloured bandages and plasters that are available so that in the event of them coming off into the food they are easily recognisable.

Any break of the skin, whether it be a scratch or cut, should be washed in warm water containing antiseptic and covered with a soft dressing and, if food handlers are involved, this should then be covered with a water-proof dressing. Any cut or abrasion may harbour *Staphylococci* bacteria and the intention is to prevent any contamination to the food through a discharge. If left uncovered, towels, utensils and equipment as well as the food, may become infected and one can imagine the consequences. Fingers are the most vulnerable part of any food handler and bandage should never be used alone but should be covered with a suitable dressing, finger stall or perhaps a rubber glove. If there is an uncontrollable discharge then the food handler must stop handling food and should immediately see a doctor.

Chapter 9

MARKETS, STALLS AND DELIVERY VEHICLES

This chapter attempts to deal with food hygiene in markets, on stalls and in delivery vehicles. In many instances it is more important to observe the highest standards of cleanliness in mobile or temporary food retailing than in fixed premises. The principal reason for this is the simple construction of, say, a market stall compared to a conventional shop building with all its modern conveniences. Modern mobile shops and delivery vehicles are built to a good standard and all three categories will be examined separately in this chapter.

As with all hygienic handling of food, common sense plays a leading part. In practice, it will be found that designing and constructing mobile premises to the highest standard will pay enormous dividends, both in terms of labour saving and sales resulting from the hygienic image which the public appreciates more and more.

A special set of regulations apply to this part of the food trade, namely the Food Hygiene (Markets, Stalls & Delivery Vehicles) Regulations, 1966, which are discussed in Chapter 1 and which should be studied by every mobile trader and salesman.

Certain regulations apply to every person engaged in handling food, whether as a stall holder, ice-cream salesman or van driver. These rules concern personal hygiene and should be familiar to readers by now. A brief reminder, however, that clothing should be clean and washable even in the depths of winter; hands should be kept clean; cuts or abrasions should be covered with waterproof dressings; no smoking or similar habits should be indulged; and all food should be handled in a hygienic manner and wrapped in clean materials.

Stalls

This term covers a wide range of situations where food is handled other than in "fixed premises", meaning shops. The traditional market stall is of wooden construction with two or four wheels, whereas the mobile ice-cream van should be constructed of aluminium, stainless steel and glass fibre/plastic laminates.

Market stalls should be constructed of impervious materials in order to make cleaning easy and efficient. Hard woods with painted finishes are commonly used, although glass fibre and metal stalls are now available. The stall must be fitted with a superstructure, because the top and three sides must be enclosed with impervious material to prevent the risk of contamination. Additionally the covering keeps the rain off in outdoor markets. The sheeting is often a lightweight plastic or durable polythene, which may be transparent to let in plenty of light. If trading is carried out during hours of darkness, then adequate artificial lighting must be provided to make sure that safe food handling is practised.

Another important rule is that every stall must conspicuously display the name and address of the person responsible for the business. This is to enable an aggrieved customer to identify the trader in the event of a complaint. Some traders have arrangements with the Health Department of the local authority whereby the stall displays the trader's name and stall number only, but this is not a universal practice.

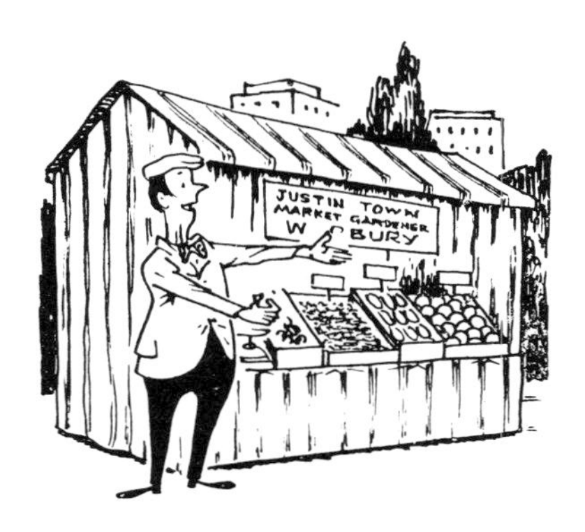

Food on or around the stall must not be placed within 45cm (18in) of the ground, unless it is protected from contamination. Dirt, dust, or even dogs could cause this at any time. Refuse should be stored in suitable bins, or other containers, and these should be emptied at least daily. Rubbish should not be allowed to accumulate on or around the stall or vehicle.

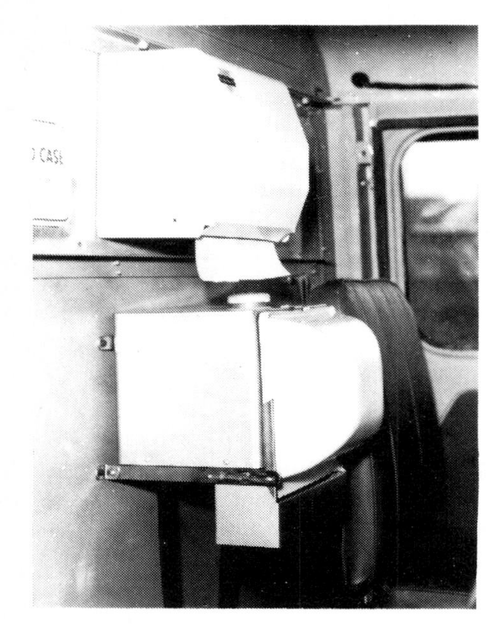

Hand washing unit in a vehicle cab (Teal Patents Ltd)

On many food stalls it is necessary to provide one or more sinks with a hot and cold water supply for washing food and equipment. If the sink is only used to wash fruit, fish or vegetables, then only cold water is required. In certain circumstances, the trader can apply to the local authority for an exemption certificate; e.g. a fruiterer or greengrocer may dispense with a sink.

Washhand basins with hot or cold running water, together with soap, towel and nailbrush to ensure hygienic handling, must also be provided for the use of food handlers.

In practice these requirements have led to various difficulties because of the nature of both stalls and vehicles. A series of small purpose-built units are manufactured for mobile traders. They comprise a small insulated storage tank which can either be filled with hot water before leaving the garage or trading base, or be connected to the vehicle's radiator to provide heated water.

In the case of open air markets, the owner or local authority usually provides public conveniences to which the stall holders can resort, and the washing facilities therein can be used. Notwithstanding this, however, one of the big problems is that hands can get very dirty from handling coins. This is why washing facilities should be readily available on all stalls.

There is such a wide variety of food being sold from stalls and vehicles that it is difficult to generalise, but the basic intention is that stalls and vehicles should endeavour to comply with the same standards as shop premises. After all, the risk of contamination is equally great, if not greater.

There are a few types of mobile trader who deserve special consideration because of their potential threat to human health if poor hygienic standards are allowed to exist. We refer to the ice-cream salesman, the hot dog stall and the roadside refreshment stall in particular. These forms of mobile food vending tend to attract their fair share of criticism, largely due to the unattractive appearance of some of their equipment. The major problems, however, relate to the types of food being handled and sold. In particular, the lack of adequate facilities for storing the perishable products at a safe temperature produces the consequent danger of unhygienic or unsound food being sold to the public. Meat products and ice-cream are two of the most likely foods to be connected with food poisoning. (See Chapter 2).

Another potentially dangerous food group is shellfish, which are commonly sold from stalls outside public houses. The problem lies principally with those shellfish which are contaminated before they are harvested. Although regular sampling by the health authorities endeavours to prevent them being sold, there are numerous examples of prawns, shrimps, cockles, whelks, mussels and oysters being the cause of illness and even death amongst human beings. The problem is that no-one can detect bacterial contamination without laboratory examination, so that stallholders must ensure strict hygienic practices and equipment to prevent or reduce the risk of serious trouble.

Once again it must be emphasised that the presentation and appearance of any food retailer's equipment and sales staff produce the image which will create success. Public awareness of hygiene standards these days will readily result in dirty premises losing trade.

A special mention must also be made of food hygiene at open air funtions where large numbers of the public attend. These range from football and cricket grounds to open air theatres, motor racing circuits, fairs and rallies, fêtes and gymkhanas, barbecues and wedding receptions — the list is endless. Unfortunately the risks are just the same and the need for vigilance even greater, because the problems of providing constant hot water and drainage, electricity and all the normal sevices are often a major headache.

Unfortunately one often finds bar staff in the marquee trying to wash dirty glasses in cold water (the lipstick just won't come off!) and food being prepared on trestle tables set up in a field full of cow pats! Apart from the lack of adequate hygiene, the working conditions for the stall can be very primitive (with a chemical closet tucked away in a corner if you are lucky). This is one aspect of catering and food retailing which needs closer scrutiny by the Health Department in most areas of the country. There is no excuse for lower standards of food handling at these functions. It is up the organisers or proprietors of the businesses to ensure the highest standards.

A question arises from time to time in connection with voluntary bodies and organisations, schools, Women's Institutes, Cricket and Rugby Clubs, who inquire whether they have to comply with the law when handling or selling food to raise money for their funds or charities. The answer is a definite "YES", because the law defines a food business as "whether selling for profit or not". This particular requirement also encompasses housewives who cook cakes and dishes at home for subsequent sale at clubs and jumble sales. The most unsatisfactory feature of using the domestic kitchen for commercial food preparation on any scale is that the kitchen is rarely designed for catering as such. The same sink may be used for babies' nappies, the vegetables, the food preparation and the washing-up. The risk of cross-contamination is very real and is even greater with the presence of domestic pets.

Having observed a large cross-section of domestic premises at close quarters, the authors are forced to the conclusion that not every housewife would be proud of her kitchen!

Delivery vehicles

Modern food marketing techniques invariably involve the packaging of products at the point of manufacture so that many foodstuffs are transported in protective wrappings. The nature of the product determines the type of wrapping: metal can, rigid polythene carton, vacuum package, cardboard box, waxed paper container, glass jar, plastic tub, aluminium foil, or polystyrene carton. It also determines the method of transport, namely refrigerated lorry, articulated freezer container or plain van. Naturally these variables will affect the design, construction and equipping of the vehicle, although the common theme will be of using suitable materials to provide a hygienic, easily-cleansed interior.

All fleet transport vehicles are built to high standards using stainless steel, alloyed aluminium or galvanised mild-steel welded plate. Non-slip flooring is fitted and the body is carefully insulated to prevent extremes of

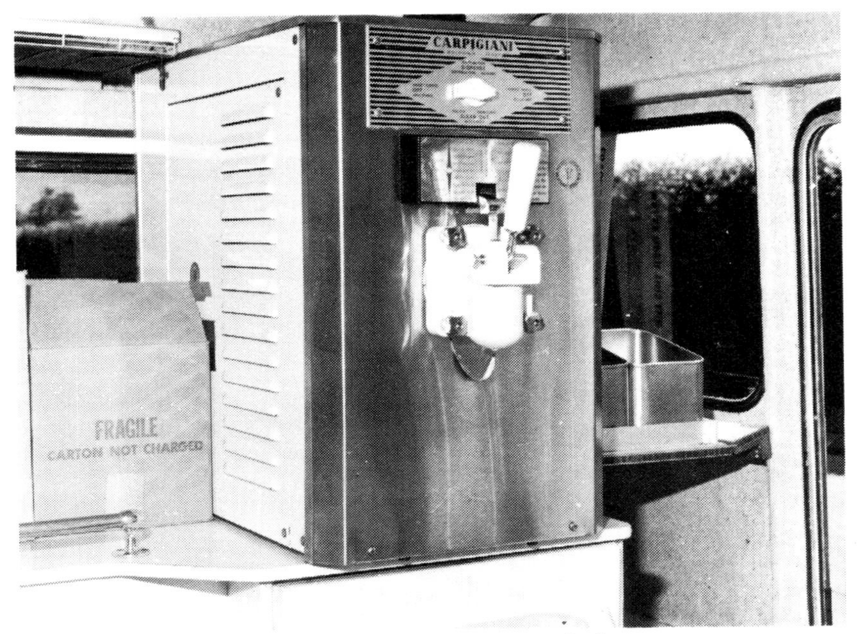

A well-equipped mobile vehicle (T. Walls (Ice-cream) Ltd)

temperature occurring. Special attention must be paid to vehicles transporting frozen foods because the temperature of the vehicle must be maintained to match that of the cold store and the freezer unit into which the food is to be placed. Normally a temperature range of —20°C to —5°C (—7° to 22°F) is encountered. The less exposure there is to fluctuating temperatures, the longer the shelf life of the commodity.

Meat, bread and fresh vegetables are the most common foods still transported with little or no outer wrapping to offer protection against contamination. With meat and bakery products in particular, it is therefore important that the vehicles and containers are kept clean and that the food is carefully handled on and off the vehicle. Personnel are required to wear clean, washable overclothing, including headwear in the case of meat carriers, and to observe the hygiene rules listed above.

To assist staff to maintain personal cleanliness when handling food on vehicles, especially for direct retail sale, certain vehicles must be provided with a washhand basin, a supply of hot and cold water, soap, towel and nail brush. Such vehicles include ice-cream vans and mobile shops (unless selling entirely wrapped food).

Exemptions are allowed for delivery vehicles, provided hand-washing facilities are available at each premises at which collections or deliveries are made. This also applies to bread vans. Ideally, all vehicles should be provided with washing facilities for the delivery-men.

First aid equipment should be carried on all vehicles and in the case of mobile shops at least one sink with hot and cold water supplies should be provided to enable equipment to be kept clean. The owner's name and address should be conspicuously displayed on the vehicle.

A planned routine of cleaning food vehicles should be carried out every day, using plenty of hot soapy water followed by careful rinsing with clean water. A combined detergent/disinfectant can be used to advantage as an alternative to live steam for removing grease, fat and dirt.

Vending machines

Perhaps this is a little out of place in this chapter but, nonetheless, it is a form of food retailing which is frequently encountered today. There are vending machines capable of serving most types of food, from hot beverages to instant hot meals; consequently the hygiene of the equipment needs to be given high priority.

Most modern vending machines have been designed and constructed to high standards with efficient cleansing in mind, thus quality materials such as stainless steel are often used. Automatic cut-outs are incorporated in the machine to prevent sales continuing if the machine overheats, overflows or fails to function safely. Machines are designed to prevent access by vermin or pests and food containers are covered to prevent risk of contamination.

Cleaning instructions are normally displayed on the machine and should be closely followed. Machines should be cleaned daily. Records should be kept with the machine, detailing the date and time of cleaning. Liberal quantities of hot water with a detergent, or combined detergent/disinfectant solution, should be used to cleanse all parts of the machine liable to be in contact with food. Particular attention should be paid to tubes and containers used for milk, water and liquid beverages; water tanks should also be emptied and refilled with fresh water.

Particular care must be taken to ensure that the machine is working at the correct temperature to keep the food in prime condition. Ice-cream temperatures must not rise above —2°C (28°F); meat products, cheese, dry beverages, etc. must stay below 10°C (50°F). Careful stock rotation and ordering is also important when selling fresh perishable food from a machine. All food should therefore be coded with the appropriate "sell by" or "death" date. Failure to observe these basic hygiene rules will result in reduced sales and, more importantly, the risk of bacterial infection from the unclean parts of the machine on which food particles are allowed to accumulate. Many modern designs incorporate "one trip" parts so that sterile materials are fitted at least daily on all parts of the machine in contact with food.

Finally, don't forget to empty the adjacent litter bin frequently. This can be the biggest deterrent to sales, if left to overflow and become unsightly.

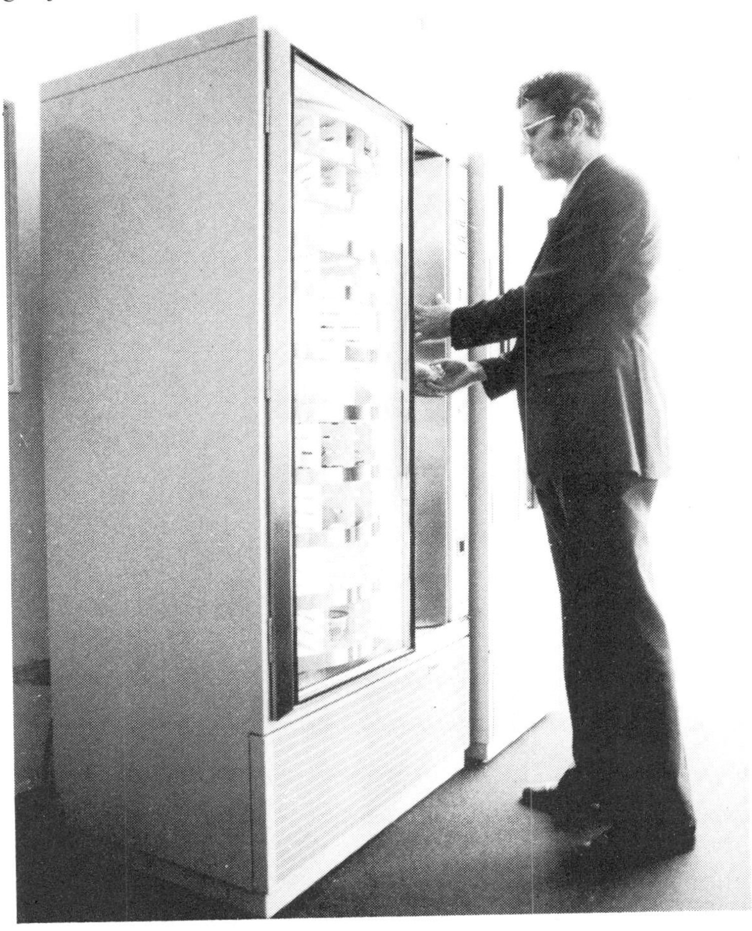

A large automatic vending machine

Chapter 10

HEALTH, SAFETY AND WELFARE

At first glance this chapter may seem a little out of place in a book about food hygiene. A closer study, however, will show how inextricably the two subjects are linked when one considers, for example, that the "No Smoking" rule to prevent contamination will also reduce the risk of a fire and the clean, grease-free floor will reduce the chances of an accident to a member of the staff.

The Factories Acts and the Offices, Shops and Railway Premises Act have been with us for a number of years and have set standards giving many employees reasonable working conditions. The Health & Safety at Work Act, 1974, introduced a new concept whereby everyone became involved from the employer and the employee, the self-employed and the manufacturer to the supplier and the general public. Many premises and their employees were protected for the first time by this Act, which many experts consider to be one of the most important pieces of legislation to be passed this century.

The Act involves everyone from the Managing Director to the pot boy, and each person has a responsibility to ensure that his or her actions do not put either him, her or anyone else in danger. The employer must issue a health and safety policy statement to all staff indicating the management's attitude to these matters, and staff must receive adequate training for their jobs. Suppliers of machinery and materials must ensure that these are safe to use and instructions are issued on safe working methods. It is illegal to supply machinery without proper guarding, e.g. food slicers, but the Act places the onus on an employee to use the equipment properly. If the guard has been removed, then the employee may not only have a nasty accident but may be fined in Court as well. Suitable protective clothing should be available in certain situations, and this is another link with food hygiene and the need to wear clean, washable garments.

A fundamental concept of the legislation is that the premises must be a safe place not only for the staff but also for the customers. This means that the building itself should be sound and that furniture, flooring, machinery and equipment have to be safe to use and maintained in that condition. One company has been prosecuted because a window fell inwards on to a customer! Adequate fire precautions, equipment and emergency instructions are naturally required in all buildings as is the provision of first aid equipment and nursing staff in large organisations.

Other fundamental concepts of the Act are the emphasis on consulting employees and organising training to ensure that staff know how to work safely and what hazards and dangers may confront them. Sprained muscles, especially back-ache, are a very common occurrence due to incorrect lifting, but how many people have been taught the simple rules of correct lifting? The food industry is particularly prone to accidents such as cuts, burns, scalds and worse, so it is essential that staff are properly trained in correct working methods and practices to reduce the risk of injury to a minimum. Young people at the start of their careers are particularly in need of adequate instruction before they acquire bad habits and attitudes. Senior staff have a particular responsibility to ensure that safety rules are obeyed and that hazardous premises and practices are immediately corrected.

What is meant by health, safety and welfare in practice?

Health

This subject has already been examined in Chapter 2, dealing with food poisoning, in which it was explained how food handlers suffering from intestinal disorders, ear, nose or throat infections and skin infections can spread bacteria and ultimately cause infection in other people. Persons suffering from typhoid, paratyphoid, dysentery, food poisoning and other specified infectious diseases are prohibited from handling food until medically cleared to resume work.

Good health is of paramount importance to all persons engaged in handling food, and it is in the employers' interests to ensure that their staffs are given reasonable facilities to achieve and maintain good health. Enlightened companies offer special medical facilities and schemes whereby employees can obtain specialist medical advice outside the

National Health Service system. Many large factories and departmental stores employ trained nursing staff, including consultant doctors, to supervise the health of employees. Such a service may include compulsory examination of employees at regular intervals to monitor the risk of infection. Every food business must provide and maintain a sufficient supply of first aid equipment as required by law. (See Chapter 1, page 6).

There are a number of industrial diseases, including dermatitis and bronchitis, which can be contracted in food premises like flour mills. The wearing of protective clothing, such as face masks, may well be necessary to reduce the risk of industrial injury or ill-health.

Damage to hearing is another health risk caused through employees not being provided with, or not wearing, ear muffs or earplugs when working at or near noisy machinery. Checks can be made to assess the noise levels and measures taken to sound-proof or insulate the offending equipment in many instances. Exposure to noise causes a gradual deterioration in the individual's power of hearing which is often not appreciated until serious deafness is a fact.

The eyesight can be damaged as a result of either inadequate artificial lighting or unshaded lights which cause glare. Both of these could and should be corrected by lighting consultants. It is not commonly realised that whereas natural sunlight gives light readings of around 5,000 lux, the average artificial lighting in a building is in the order of 500 lux. The eyes adjust to the poorer light intensity, but eyestrain frequently occurs and there is no substitute for sufficient artificial lighting.

While on the subject of health, it is perhaps opportune to remember that smoking is not only a bad habit from the food contamination and fire safety angles, but also because of the proven risk of lung diseases, particularly cancer, which are associated with cigarette smoking.

Safety

This subject has already been explored in various aspects, but one cannot underestimate the inherent dangers which are encountered daily in food premises. Dangers will range from slippery floors caused by grease and water in the kitchen or over-zealous polishing of the parquet flooring in the dining-room, to hot-plates, ovens, knives, dumb waiters, carbon dioxide gas cylinders, trolleys, refrigeration equipment — the list is endless. Safety rules must be obeyed in everyone's interest, and nobody should be expected to risk injury or even death through the use of dangerous equipment or practices.

In larger organisations, there will be designated Safety Officers with special responsibility for all aspects of safety. They will be assisted by managers, supervisors and other responsible staff who have been trained to pay particular attention to safety within their department, shift or team.

Fire causes millions of pounds worth of damage in Britain each year and many lives are lost. The individual's knowledge of the fire exits and fire drill are particularly important, and regular practices are extremely valuable. There is less likelihood of panic if the routine is established. People will also realise the importance of fire check doors and not wedge them open, if it is explained that deaths are more often due to asphyxiation from smoke than from the fire itself.

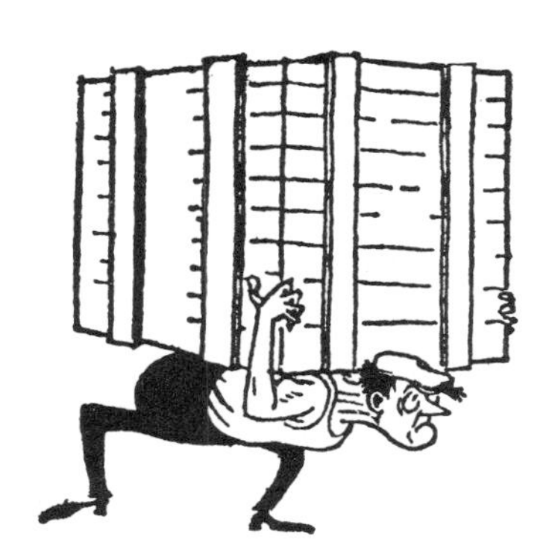

Correct lifting methods . . .

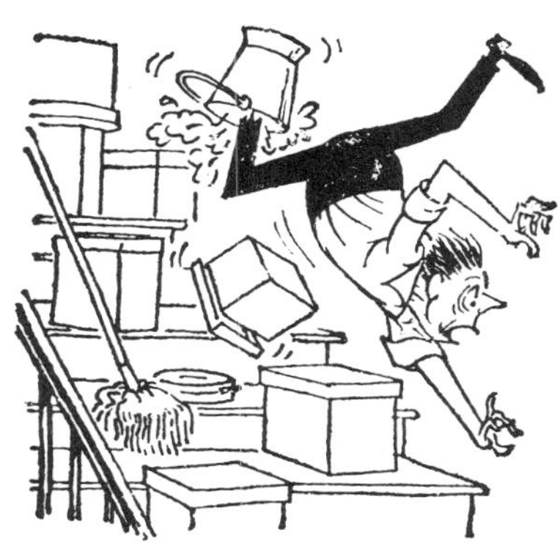

uncluttered stairs . . .

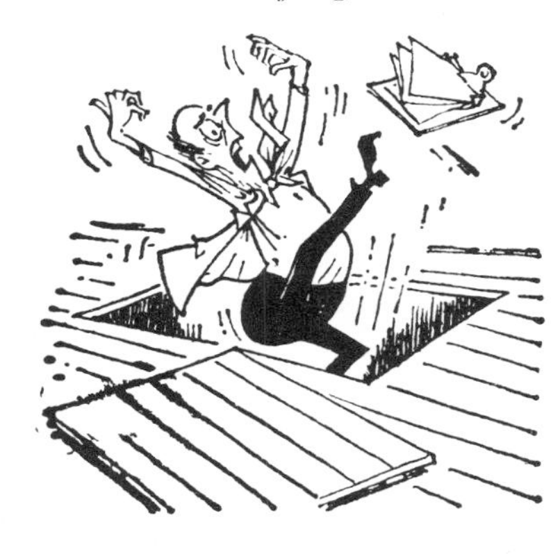

unguarded openings . . .

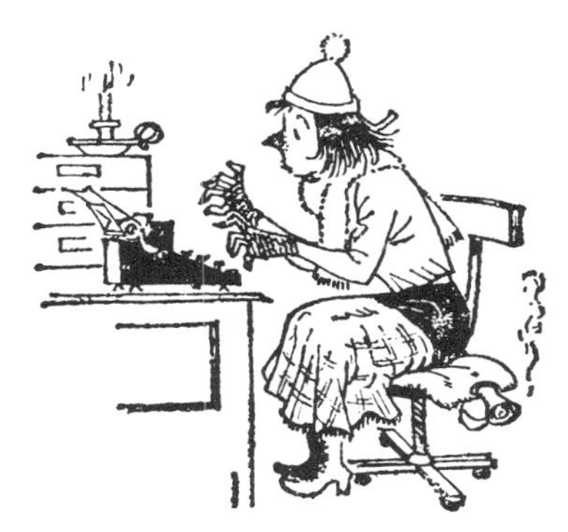

adequate heating . . .

. . . are among the responsibilities of management and staff alike under the new concepts of the important Health and Safety at Work, etc, Act, 1974

Welfare

This is one area where widely differing standards are adopted in industry. Some companies realise the advantages in providing facilities and amenities for staff, whereas others let staff fend for themselves. Common examples of such facilities would be staff canteens, concessionary shops, sports facilities and medical schemes, but some companies also offer staff hairdressing and manicuring facilities — even sauna baths are known to exist for the weary employee!

On a more mundane level, there are legal requirements governing the provision of basic welfare facilities such as sanitary accommodation, facilities for the disposal of sanitary and surgical dressings, drinking water supplies, washing facilities, cloakrooms, the provision of suitable equipment, seating, the maintenance of sufficient heating (generally 16°C/60°F minimum), the provision of adequate space in which to work, and the maintenance of clean working conditions and premises.

Enforcement of the Legislation

The duties of the two main Inspectorates currently overlap in many premises. An attempt has been made to clarify the situation, to split the types of food premises up to reduce the amount of dual inspection, and it is likely that the local authorities' Environmental Health Departments will be responsible not only for food hygiene regulations but also the Health & Safety at Work Act and Regulations in most classes of food premises: food shops, hotels, restaurants, canteens, and departmental stores. There will be some food factories, however, where the Health & Safety Inspectors (Factory Inspectors) will still be responsible for enforcing the Act and the Health Officer will also visit the premises under the Food and Hygiene Regulations.

Because of the additional responsibilities placed on enforcing Officers by the Health & Safety at Work Act, it is possible that routine inspections will take much longer to complete. The management and the staff can demand to accompany the Officer on his/her inspection and to receive copies of any subsequent report which may be made following the inspection.

If contraventions of the Act are observed, the Inspector can choose which course of action to take. If the defect is likely to present an imminent risk of serious injury, then an Immediate Prohibition Notice can be served on the owner or proprietor. This means that the machine or procedure must cease until it is rendered safe. Alternatively a Deferred Prohibition Notice may be served if there is, or will be, a possible risk of serious personal injury. A third course would be to serve an Improvement Notice. This could be served where a contravention is found which needs to be remedied within a specified period of time.

Finally, a prosecution may be considered if previous written or verbal warnings have been ignored and/or the contravention of the Act is so serious that the enforcing Officer feels that a fine is the only method of drawing the offender's attention to the need to take health, safety and welfare matters seriously. Inspectors always carry a means of identification, which has to be produced on request, and are entitled to enter any premises at any reasonable time without prior warning. Police officers are entitled to accompany the Inspector, who is also empowered to take samples of materials and equipment, photographs and to make sound recordings, if necessary.

If a person feels that a notice has been unjustly served on him/her, there is an appeals procedure to an Industrial Tribunal within 21 days of the service of the notice.

Good management and business practice suggests that staff will not work efficiently if health, safety and welfare conditions are below standard. Unsatisfactory premises which create hazards to the customers or publicity following a prosecution will be bad for business. It must make sense to promote a bright, safe, hygienic image at all times.

The following check list has been prepared as a summary of the principal health, safety and welfare requirements which every commercial company should meet.

HEALTH AND SAFETY CHECK LIST

1. Is the accident book kept up to date?
2. Is the first aid kit properly stocked and easily accessible to staff?
3. Have the staff received first aid training?
4. What action would you take in the event of a serious accident to a member of the staff or a customer?
5. Are all staff provided with suitable protective clothing for their various jobs?
6. Is all equipment fitted with proper guards to prevent accidents?
7. Are instructions displayed and staff trained to operate equipment in a safe manner?
8. Are regular inspections of all equipment undertaken by a competent engineer or electrician?
9. Have staff been instructed in the action to be taken in the event of fire; is suitable fire fighting equipment readily available?
10. Are the emergency services telephone numbers clearly displayed — e.g., fire, ambulance, police, gas, electricity, fire, water?
11. Are the staff cloakroom facilities adequate and regularly cleaned and inspected?
12. Do you know how to contact the local Environmental Health Officer for advice?

Chapter 11

HEALTH EDUCATION

The days when health education was the sole responsibility of the nurse, environmental health officer, doctor or teacher have long since gone, and it is generally accepted that all food handlers and especially those in a supervisory capacity have an important part to play. As it implies, health education is the process whereby food handlers are advised, informed or educated into realising why certain practices are necessary in food premises. Outbreaks of food poisoning are invariably the result of faulty food handling rather than faulty premises.

Staff may be educated in a number of ways but the most effective and, therefore, the most important is teaching by example. This example must be set from the top by management and supervisory staff and can only be achieved if they themselves have clean and tidy dress and they themselves practice good personal hygiene. Junior staff are much more likely to take note of how their seniors perform their duties, than by receiving any amount of advisory literature. While the latter is important, it should be regarded only as a supplementary aid.

Newly engaged staff, and this particularly applies to new recruits to the industry, need some basic training in the particular business involved; whether it be restaurant catering, factory catering or a retail supermarket, for each presents its own special needs and problems. Staff in all types of food premises, however, need a sound basic knowledge of food hygiene and while much can be achieved through an in-service training programme, most benefit can be gained by attending a specialist course on the subject.

Courses are often organised by local authority environmental health

PLEASE WASH YOUR HANDS
請洗手
PLEASE DO NOT SMOKE
SI PREGA
DI NON FUMARE
Eaton
PLEASE WASH YOUR HANDS
LAVEN SUS MANOS
POR FAVOR
EATON ENTERPRISES, P.O. Box 34, Walton-on-Thames, Surrey, KT12 3JR
Sp.
PLEASE DO NOT SMOKE
請勿吸煙

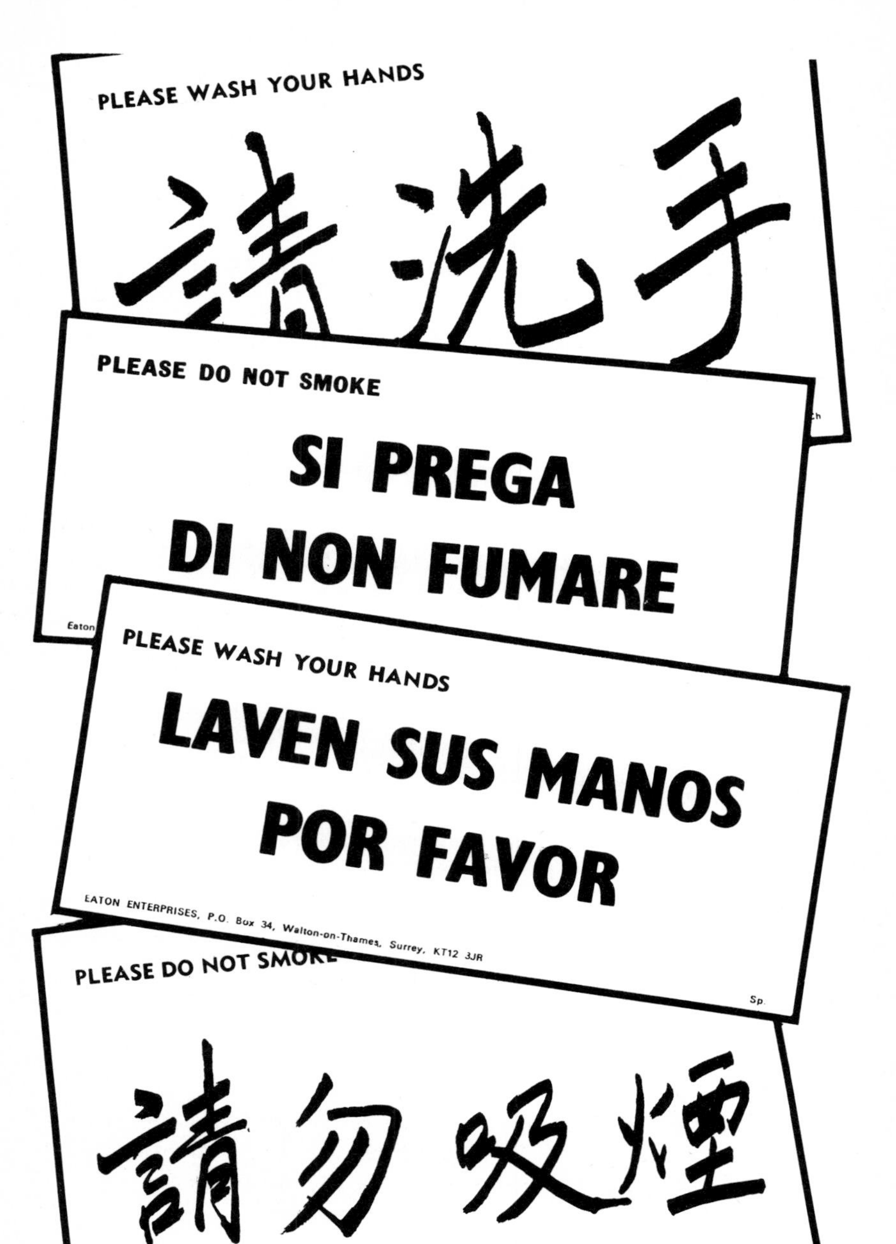

Messages in foreign langauages are useful aids in the battle for cleanliness (Eaton Publications)

departments, either on their own or in conjunction with a local technical college. Management should endeavour to send all staff on such a course.

One of the advantages of attending a course is that while the food handler may know what his responsibilities are, it is important that he should know why they are necessary. Knowing that you have to wash your hands after using the lavatory is one thing but knowing *why* is another. Once aware of the reasons, the handler is much more likely to observe the requirement.

Although the manager or supervisor must ultimately be responsible for food hygiene standards in any food premises, many firms have appointed a member of the staff as hygiene officer or assistant. Their job is to give basic training to staff and to keep an eye on standards generally. Such an appointment can more than justify itself and, indeed, some of the larger firms have made full-time appointments for this purpose.

Very often, environmental health officers will organise short courses on the premises, especially where numbers justify it.

Again management should consult their local authority to see if this is possible. The organisation of food hygiene courses will depend on a number of factors, not least amongst these being the amount of staff time which can be spared and the amount of time the local environmental health officer can offer. In the knowledge that whatever time is spent in training is time well spent, the following two programmes are put forward as suggestions for in-service training courses.

Six Week — One Hour a Week — Food Hygiene Course

[*This is most suitable for supervisory staff*]

1. Introduction to food hygiene and food poisoning.
2. Personal hygiene.
3. The food handler and the law.
4. The design and maintenance of food premises.
5. Storage of food.
6. Summary of course and general forum.

Three Week — One Hour a Week — Course for Food Handlers

[*This is a basic programme for middle and lower level personnel or those who are unable to attend the longer course for lack of time*]

1. Introduction to food hygiene and food poisoning.
2. Personal hygiene.
3. The design and maintenance of food premises/the storage of food.

A number of suitable films are available from various film libraries or private firms. Advice on the choice of film is always available from your local environmental health department.

Many people engaged in the catering industry have obtained qualifications ranging from university degrees in food and nutrition to diplomas in food technology. The Hotel and Catering Industry Training Board is particularly active in promoting training at all levels. It is generally recognised that, however good the qualifications may be, everyone benefits from receiving further training from time to time on new developments and trends.

"Familiarity breeds contempt". This is a favourite saying which has stood the test of time. Constant reminders of food hygiene and safety responsibilities are necessary; these can be both verbal from managers or in the form of posters and notices. Short sharp messages are best because these are quickly read, whereas detailed instructions often take too long to read and do not catch the attention of the worker.

Food Hygiene (General) Regulations 1970

Points for food handlers to remember . . .

1. Hands must be clean.
2. Overclothing must be clean and washable.
3. Cuts or abrasions must be covered with a suitable waterproof dressing.
4. Spitting is prohibited.
5. The use of snuff, tobacco or other smoking mixture is prohibited.
6. In the event of a food handler feeling ill, the employer should be notified and the doctor consulted.
7. Hands must be washed after using the lavatory.

Further details in connection with the Food Hygiene (General) Regulations 1970 may be obtained from the local Public Health Department.

Sort, sharp messages are the most effective!

While training by example and attendance at specialist courses can be most valuable, a large amount of literature is available to assist the food handler in understanding his responsibilities.

The Food Hygiene Regulations, 1970, are available in a simplified form and in various languages. If a food handler is to conform with the law, then he should have some idea of what the law says in the first place. Many local authorities distribute copies of the Regulations and other advisory literature free to food handlers while some firms purchase supplies themselves. Whichever the case, it is important for each food firm to have some advisory literature available covering the basic requirements and quite definitely every manager and supervisor should have a copy of the Food Hygiene Regulations as a constant companion.

BIBLIOGRAPHY

Bender, Arnold E., *The Facts of Food;* Oxford University Press, 1975
Dewberry, Elliot B., *Food Poisoning;* Leonard Hill (Books) Ltd, 1959
Ford, B.J., *Microbiology and Food,* Northwood Publications Ltd, 1971
Graham-Rack, Barry and Raymond Binstead, *Hygiene in Food Manufacturing and Handling;* Food Trade Press, 1973
Grundy, Elizabeth, *Dangerous People;* Spectator Publications Ltd and IZAL Ltd

Thought for Food; City of Canterbury, 1976
Clean Catering: Handbook on Premises, Equipment and Practices for the Promotion of Hygiene in Food Establishments; H.M.S.O., 1972
Microbiological Aspects of Food Hygiene; World Health Organisation

Robers, Diane, *Observations on procedures for thawing and spit-roasting frozen dressed chickens and post-cooking care and storage;* Journal of Hygiene (1972), Cambridge

APPENDIX

In order to test your knowledge of the basic principles of food hygiene, see if you can answer the questions listed in Appendix 1. If you score 18-20 marks in each set you are excellent; 13-17 marks you are average; 9-12 marks you are below average; and if you score only 1-8 marks — you should reread the book!

Questions: Set 1

1. Does freezing food kill bacteria?
2. Within which temperature range do bacteria most readily multiply?
3. Name the three most common types of bacteria likely to cause food poisoning.
4. Name three foods which are most likely to be associated with food poisoning.
5. Above what temperature should hot food be kept before serving?
6. What is the most likely cause of contamination during food preparation?
7. How should meat pies be stored over night?
8. Why are flies such harmful insects?
9. What would you do if a rat or mouse has been seen on your premises?
10. What is meant by the term "a healthy carrier"?
11. Why is the date coding of food so important?
12. Is the use of sawdust or cardboard on a slippery floor a good idea?
13. Why should cooked meat and raw food be kept separate?
14. Should domestic pets be allowed in food rooms?
15. Why shouldn't a food handler smoke while handling open food?
16. Why might tea towels be dangerous?
17. What are the advantages of stainless steel over wood in a kitchen?
18. What is meant by the term "cross contamination"?
19. Why is it important to wash hands after using the lavatory?
20. Why should food be handled as little as possible?

Now be bold and turn to page 130 for the answers!

Questions: Set 2

1. Which bacteria is commonly found in the ear, nose and throat region?
2. What are the physical conditions necessary for the growth of bacteria?
3. By what method do bacteria multiply?
4. What is the incubation period of *Salmonella* bacteria?
5. How should refuse be stored?
6. What is the difference between a detergent and a disinfectant?
7. What method would you recommend for hand drying?
8. What is meant by the term "safe food"?
9. Why are oysters and mussels a potential danger to public health?
10. How often should a slicing machine be cleaned?
11. How should ice-cream servers be kept when not in use?
12. Name the equipment that mixes a measured dose of detergent with water on a tap.
13. Name three methods of preserving food.
14. Why is good lighting necessary in food premises?
15. What causes a can to be "blown"?
16. If you have some "suspicious" food, who would you contact to examine it?
17. What must a first-aid kit contain in a food premises?
18. Food containers are best made from .... ?
19. Why should frozen poultry be thoroughly thawed before cooking?
20. Do you have a copy of the Food Hygiene Regulations?

Answers on page 131.

Answers to Set 1

1. It can kill some.
2. 10-63°C (50-145°F).
3. *Salmonella; Staphylococci; Clostridium welchii.*
4. Meat; fish; gravy; cream; eggs; milk.
5. 63°C (145°F).
6. Dirty hands.
7. In a refrigerator.
8. They can carry dirt and disease.
9. Check all stock for contamination and contact a specialist pest control firm immediately.
10. A person who carries disease bacteria but who does not show the symptons of that disease.
11. It enables the retailer to use older stock first.
12. No; because it can harbour bacteria.
13. Because of the danger of cross contamination: the transfer of bacteria from the uncooked meat to the cooked meat.
14. No.
15. Besides the possibility of ash falling in the food, there is the danger of harmful bacteria being transferred from the mouth by the fingers to the food.
16. If dirty, they can contaminate otherwise clean utensils.
17. It is impervious and can be readily cleaned.
18. It is the transfer of bacteria from one food to another through contact with a common piece of equipment; e.g. a knife or cutting board.
19. To remove bacteria from the hands; bearing in mind that lavatory paper is porous.
20. Hands are a common source of contamination.

Answers to Set 2

1. *Staphylococci.*
2. Food; temperature; moisture; time.
3. Binary fission.
4. 12-24 hours.
5. In well-constructed containers with tight-fitting lids.
6. A detergent only cleans; a disinfectant destroys bacteria.
7. Continuous roller towel; disposable paper towels; hot air.
8. Food that can be eaten without causing illness.
9. They are grown in estuaries which may become polluted with sewage.
10. Between different foods and at the end of each day.
11. In a disinfectant solution which should be regularly changed.
12. Tap proportioner.
13. Heat; freezing; drying; addition of chemicals.
14. Enables workers to see what they are doing and shows up any dirt.
15. The creation of gas caused through a decomposition of the food. Acid food attacking metal to liberate gas (faulty canning).
16. The local environmental health officer.
17. Bandages; waterproof dressings; antiseptic.
18. A smooth, impervious material such as stainless steel, plastic or aluminium.
19. To eliminate the possibility of a frozen area remaining in the middle which would prevent adequate cooking throughout.
20. If not, why not?

INDEX